ANN LOUISE GITTLEMAN'S

GUIDE TO THE

40/30/30 PHENOMENON

Ann Louise Gittleman, M.S., C.N.S.

Contemporary Books

Chicago   New York   San Francisco   Lisbon   London   Madrid   Mexico City
Milan   New Delhi   San Juan   Seoul   Singapore   Sydney   Toronto

Library of Congress Cataloging-in-Publication Data

Gittleman, Ann Louise.
    Ann Louise Gittleman's guide to the 40/30/30 phenomenon / Ann Louise Gittleman
       p. cm.
    Includes bibliographical references and index.
    ISBN 0-658-01659-8 (alk. paper)
     1. Reducing diets—Recipes.   I. Title: Guide to the 40/30/30 phenomenon.

RM222.2 .G538 2001
613.2'5—dc21

2001038350

Contemporary Books

A Division of The McGraw·Hill Companies

1 2 3 4 5 6 7 8 9 10   AGM/AGM   10 9 8 7 6 5 4 3 2 1

ISBN 0-658-01659-8

This book was set in Janson by Laurie Young
Printed and bound by Quebecor Martinsburg

Cover design by Mike Stromberg / The Great American Art Co.

McGraw-Hill books are available at special quantity discounts to use as premiums and sales promotions, or for use in corporate training programs. For more information, please write to the Director of Special Sales, Professional Publishing, McGraw-Hill, Two Penn Plaza, New York, NY 10121-2298. Or contact your local bookstore.

This book is printed on acid-free paper.

CONTENTS

CONTENTS

ACKNOWLEDGMENTS

IT IS MY PLEASURE TO ACKNOWLEDGE PETER HOFFMAN, Phyllis Herman, and Ann Castro for their assistance with this project. I especially wish to thank Rena Copperman, who is an impeccable editor blessed with patience and perseverance—my kind of gal!

The entire ALG, Inc., team was very supportive throughout the creative and researching process for this updated 40/30/30 edition. My sincere appreciation to Stuart Gittleman, Krystie Gummer, and Laura Tengelsen.

Finally, I am grateful to my friend and colleague Dr. Barry Sears for pioneering the 40/30/30 concept in the first place.

INTRODUCTION:
THE NEW EATING EQUATION

THE WORD *PHENOMENON* IS INDEED A FITTING DESCRIPTION for the 40/30/30 nutrition program. Since this program consists of eating 40 percent carbohydrate, 30 percent protein, and 30 percent fat, you can be sure of getting the right nutrient balance that's vital for metabolism, blood sugar, and your overall well-being.

Created by my colleague and friend Barry Sears, Ph.D., this program was first popularized in Dr. Sears's first megaseller *The Zone: A Dietary Road Map to Lose Weight Permanently*. Although initially developed to treat heart disease and diabetes, permanent weight loss became its biggest claim to fame. Dr. Sears has since written seven other books about the Zone.

I was personally gratified to see the 40/30/30 approach so widely received because it embraces the same nutritional principles and concepts that I have championed and written about for many years in books such as *Beyond Pritikin* and *Eat Fat, Lose Weight*. I think you'll find my *Guide to the 40/30/30 Phenomenon* to be a great companion to these books and to the Zone experience.

No doubt about it—the Zone-based 40/30/30 diet is indeed a phenomenon! A phenomenon—because this latest diet wave has dramatically turned the tables on conventional nutritionists and dietitians with its emphasis on protein and fat and reduction in carbohydrates. A phenomenon—because of its extraordinary popularity among world-class athletes, movie stars, diabetics, and individuals all across America. But most of all, the 40/30/30 program is a phenomenon because after so many years of low-fat, high–complex carbohydrate dietary failures . . . it works. The 40/30/30 phenomenon is a user-friendly eating plan for anyone who wants to achieve peak performance, increase energy, enhance mental focus, control blood sugar, achieve long-term hunger satisfaction, and lose weight effortlessly in the process.

It's no wonder this revolutionary diet equation continues to make its mark amidst today's "diet wars." People everywhere—from celebrities to your next-door neighbors—are continually trying myriad diet regimens in hopes of winning that proverbial battle of the bulge. But these other approaches and even the theories behind them are short-lived and unscientific. And even more worrisome, they tend to raise some serious health concerns.

The good news is the 40/30/30 plan is not only healthy for long-term health, but satisfying as well. Protein power is back on our menus, plus the taste and health benefits of quality fats—without the guilt. In addition, this nutritionally sound program teaches us that there's more to watch than refined, white flour carbohydrates. Certain highly touted complex carbohydrates (potatoes, pasta, and cereals, for example) should also be consumed in moderation. Why? These high-glycemic (fast-acting) carbohydrates raise insulin—a fat-storage hormone (more about this in Chapter 3).

Simply put, lowered insulin levels mean that the body won't store as much fat after food has been metabolized to glucose or sugar. Moreover, we can better access stored body fat for energy as well as ward off hunger because our own blood sugar is on an even keel. Since this program is based upon clinical studies with athletes, diabetics, and people who wanted to lose weight at such prestigious institutions as Pepperdine University and Sansum Medical Research Foundation in Santa Barbara, California, we can feel confident in adopting it as a way of life.

Athletes in particular should take note. Harvard's Marcus Elliott, M.D., believes that if you want to burn body fat, the 40/30/30 program is significantly superior to the high-carbohydrate, low-fat approach. Dr. Elliott supervised a clinical study at the Sports Institute of South Africa with the world-renowned exercise physiologist Dr. Tim Noakes. The study involved trained cyclists who were monitored via blood workups and body parameters. Dr. Elliott concluded the following facts after the study was completed:

- The higher-protein regimen enabled the subjects to use significantly more fat for energy, including stored fat, than did a high-carbohydrate intake.
- Fat utilization increased over time. At the end of the exercise trial, the high-protein group was getting 67 percent of total energy from fat while the high-carb group was getting only 46 percent—almost 50 percent more energy from fat.
- Subjects on the higher-protein diet who exercised at moderate intensity for prolonged periods found the effort significantly easier than did the carbohydrate group, as measured by the Borg scale. (This has relevance to better compliance on the higher-protein diets.)
- The higher-protein diet suppressed insulin levels more effectively than the high-carbohydrate diet, allowing for greater access to stored fat.

Yet even with such impressive research results, in some circles the 40/30/30 program is still controversial. The reduction of high-glycemic complex carbohydrates (not just the low-fiber processed ones) and the boost in protein and fat have many diet experts in an uproar. The truth may very well be, as I have hypothesized in my book *Your Body Knows Best*, that no single diet is right for every individual. Based upon the concept of biochemical individuality, the 40/30/30 program may be better suited to the "fast burner" individual who needs more protein, more fat, and less carbohydrate for optimum energy and weight control. Many fast burners have lost weight—and kept it off—on the 40/30/30 program, a good place to begin for individuals who have failed to lose weight on other diets or who have blood sugar problems.

However, traditionally trained dietitians often recommend a basic diet with 55 percent of calories from carbohydrate, 20 percent from protein, and 25 percent from fat—a regimen that has failed for far too many individuals. Since Americans have gone low fat to no fat, the number of overweight individuals has been steadily increasing. Moreover, diabetes rose in the United States by about 6 percent in 1999 in what the government called "dramatic evidence of an unfolding epidemic." The rise is blamed largely on obesity, which was up a startling 57 percent from 1991. [1]

LOW-FAT DIETS DON'T DELIVER

For the longest time, it looked like the media blitz on the dangers of dietary fats (high cholesterol levels, increased heart disease risk, obesity) was going to succeed. Relatively large numbers of Americans changed their eating habits, increasingly cutting fats from their diets. Then the bad news started to come in. Many of those who had succeeded in excluding fat from their diets developed powerful food cravings and went on eating binges that undid all the good of their restricted diet. These individuals simply substituted unlimited carbohydrates (such as bagels, fat-free yogurts, fat-free cookies, breads, crackers, and muffins) for the missing fats.

Even the most conscientious and well-informed dieters went overboard on fat-free but high-glycemic carbohydrates such as rice cakes, potatoes, corn, and whole grain bread. They simply were not aware that many of the complex carbohydrates they were consuming (similar to the processed simple carbohydrates such as white flour bagels) produced a quick rise in blood sugar levels, which in turn created high insulin levels. Elevated insulin not only blocks the body's ability to burn stored body fat for energy but also creates a rapid fall in blood sugar levels. When blood sugar levels are low, the brain (which is fueled by blood sugar) sends an urgent signal to the body for some immediate fast-acting fuel—usually in the form of more carbohydrates, from sugary snacks to soft drinks. Sadly, the low-fat adherents were fated to a continuous roller-coaster ride of blood sugar peaks and valleys.

In my first book, *Beyond Pritikin*, I wrote about many of the other symptoms I had personally observed in the low-fat, high–complex carbohydrate devotees during and after my work as the director of nutrition at the Pritikin Longevity Center in Santa Monica, California, in the early 1980s. I noted conditions such as low energy, fatigue, allergy, yeast problems, and mood swings, as well as dry skin, hair, and nails, which I believe were due in part to the lack of the essential fatty acids that only certain fats such as seeds, nuts, and oils can supply.[2]

THE MAGIC OF FLAXSEED

In fact, according to a growing number of scientific studies, flaxseed, a rich source of essential fatty acids, is loaded with weight-loss and health-promoting benefits. Flaxseed oil fans the flames of cellular metabolism, enabling the body to generate more heat and burn more calories. This amazing oil performs as a powerful fat fighter to trigger weight loss rather than weight gain. Flaxseed contains both soluble and insoluble dietary fiber. Soluble fiber is helpful in lowering carbohydrate and cholesterol absorption, whereas insoluble fiber facilitates elimination by absorbing water in the digestive tract, proving a tremendous aid in bowel-related concerns such as constipation and diverticular disease.

Flaxseed is also a plentiful plant source of lignans—powerful antioxidants that also function as plant-based estrogens. The lignan concentration is approximately 800 times greater in whole flaxseed than in other plants. Lignans are highly regarded for their cancer-fighting and antiviral properties. Due to their phytohormone benefits, lignans are valuable in helping to assuage bothersome perimenopause and menopause symptoms such as hot flashes and night sweats.

However, flaxseed has another vital property. It is the highest vegetarian source of the essential omega-3 fatty acid known as alpha-linolenic acid (ALA). Scientific evidence from proceedings of the Flax Institute reveal that flaxseed's omega-3 strength can help combat numerous health concerns, such as heart disease, angina, arthritis, multiple sclerosis, poor liver function, depression, breast cancer, lupus, slow-healing bruises and sprains, eczema, psoriasis, acne, and dry skin.[3]

But the most pronounced effect of flaxseed appears to be with the brain. Interestingly, the no-fat/high-carb trend parallels the escalating condition among both children and adults known as attention deficit hyperactivity disorder (ADHD). The lack of mental focus and an inability to sit still among ADHD individuals could well be linked to a lack of the omega-3 oils so essential to brain and eye development. The 40/30/30 plan outlined in this book is rich in these essential fats.

Over the past twenty years, researchers have conducted various studies that showed that ADHD youths were highly deficient in fatty acids.[4] Their blood actually had lower omega-3 levels than the blood of non-ADHD children. Even more revealing, these studies also consistently demonstrated that the ADHD/fatty acid–deficient youths had a propensity toward behavioral, learning, and health problems. Using the typical approaches—medication, education, and psychology—to treat them proved insufficient. I believe the missing link is sound nutrition.

Just look at these other increasingly prevalent health trends that have surfaced since the beginning of the low-fat craze:

- Heart disease rates are unchanged—still the number-one killer in the United States.

- We're fatter than ever before—more than half of all Americans are now considered overweight.
- Diabetes is up dramatically—with a 70 percent increase among people ages thirty to thirty-nine, even though type 2 diabetes used to be found only in older adults after years of unhealthy lifestyle practices.
- New health problems have appeared out of nowhere—mysterious low-grade ailments such as chronic fatigue, food sensitivities, and *Candida albicans.*
- More people are getting cancer than ever before.
- The incidence of parasites (with such exotic names as *amoeba histolytica, giardia, cryptosporidium, blastocystis homonis,* and *cyclospora*) is also on the rise. These microscopic organisms and worms thrive particularly well on sugar or concentrated sweets of all kinds. Americans have been consuming almost 150 pounds of sugar per person per year since the fat-free craze became so popular.

Hopefully, all of these undesirable health trends will begin to reverse as we learn to embrace the principles of the 40/30/30 phenomenon. Undoubtedly the 40/30/30 diet regimen, with its commonsense approach to eating in the twenty-first century, creates one of the best foundations for ensuring a balanced diet.

WHY THIS DIET?

EVERYBODY KNOWS THAT WHAT WE EAT AND DRINK affects our health. In the past few decades, the quest for health and attractive personal appearance has led people to try a succession of special diets. Some were dangerous, others merely imaginative. Most were ultimately disappointing. These diets disappointed because either they didn't work or, even when they did work, dieters could not stay on them for very long. The reason? These diets were unbalanced; thus the body began to crave the excluded foods that good health requires.

First and foremost, a diet must be balanced in order for it to work long term. Only then will food cravings be eliminated once and for all.

Until very recently, most diets had another major shortcoming. These diets took an oversimplified, out-of-body approach—that is, they didn't take into account our internal body controls. After absorbing nutrients from food, our bodies secrete hormones to control how the nutrients are utilized. Any diet that does not take into account the effect of foods on hormones is probably doomed to failure.

The 40/30/30 diet is based on the premise that eating food evokes a hormonal response. The 40/30/30 diet is a balanced diet, one that you can stay on indefinitely without hunger or food cravings. To follow this diet, you don't have to be a zealot or believe in any wild promises. You don't have to be a vegetarian or even shun all red meat. But you do have to read on.

CHAPTER 1

A BALANCED DIET

THE 40/30/30 DIET MAINTAINS THE PROPER BALANCE between carbohydrates, proteins, and fats. Thus cravings for any of these three nutrients are eliminated. This balance of nutrients is designed to switch the body into a fat-burning mode. In the diet, 40 percent of total calories are derived from carbohydrates in the form of slow-acting or low-glycemic starches, vegetables, grains, beans, and fruit. Thirty percent of calories are from unprocessed and quality fats and oils such as olive oil, flaxseed oil, nuts, and avocado. And 30 percent of calories are from lean, complete protein sources such as low-fat cottage cheese, lean red meat, poultry, seafood, fish, soy, and whey. People typically lose body fat and unhealthy weight, gain muscle mass, and raise their HDL ("good" cholesterol) levels.

Our bodies consume blood sugar as fuel for energy, but store excess fuel as body fat due to that remarkable storage hormone produced by the pancreas known as insulin. How much white sugar should our diet contain to deliver that correct level of blood sugar? The answer is: none at all.

Since all digested carbohydrates—including those from such unlikely sources as lemons and spinach—are absorbed into our bloodstream as glucose, our bodies' sugar requirements are easily met. And unfortunately easily exceeded.

Our bodies do not need any pure sugar at all, nor do they need processed carbohydrates such as white rice, white flour pasta, bagels, breads, and cereals, which raise blood sugar levels more than sugar itself. The digestion of slow-acting or low-glycemic complex carbohydrates, proteins, and fats provides an adequate supply of blood sugar. In fact, the right amount of protein and dietary fat is crucial because it slows down the entry of carbohydrates into the system and allows for extended hunger satisfaction. Dietary fat is actually the best blood sugar stabilizer, whereas protein is considered neutral.

The longings for particular foods that we so often feel when following some new diet or nutritional recommendations are indicative that what we are eating is unbalanced in some way. A balanced diet should not leave us with cravings for some food type not included. The optimal diet is one in which you do not have to use willpower to succeed because balancing the body's chemistry relieves food cravings effortlessly.

The bottom line is that too much or too little of the wrong kinds of carbohydrates, proteins, or fats can cause health problems. Here is a simple overview of our bodies' nutritional requirements:

- **Carbohydrates.** We need complex carbohydrates from starches, vegetables, legumes, whole grains, and fruits to provide fuel in the form of blood sugar for energy-burning brain and muscle activity.
- **Fats.** We need fats in the form of oils, nuts, and seeds to help balance the blood sugar level, to provide the raw materials for hormones, to assist in long-term energy, and to strengthen cell walls and mucous membranes.
- **Protein.** Protein from both lean animal and vegetable sources such as white meat poultry, fish, lean meat, low-fat cottage cheese, tofu, and whey helps with stabilizing blood sugar, promoting cell

growth and repair, hormone production, cell metabolism, bodily fluid balance, maintenance of the immune system, and digestive enzyme function.

All meals must consist of a *balance* of carbohydrates, proteins, and fats. A stable blood sugar level is one of the rewards of a balanced diet. With stable blood sugar, you have fewer health risks, extended energy, balanced moods, and greater mental focus and attention.

As an elementary, commonsense concept of nutrition, balance might not seem to be worth mentioning were it not for the fact that it is so often ignored. Living mostly on junk food, as so many Americans do, is one way to ensure an unbalanced diet. Another way is to go on a diet that restricts you from eating some of the foods your body needs to stay healthy. Carbohydrate loading by athletes is an example of knowingly eating an unbalanced diet.

When carbohydrate loading, athletes often eat a diet in which 70 percent of the calories are derived from carbohydrates, 15 percent from fats, and 15 percent from proteins. As you might expect, these dieters tend to get a quick energy boost that is followed by a lull in energy and a loss of mental concentration. It's no surprise that we often hear of marathon runners "hitting the wall," cyclists who "bonk," and tennis players who "lose their focus."

For sustained physical and mental effort, whether in a competitive sport or daily life, a far better ratio has proved to be 40, 30, and 30 percent carbohydrates, fats, and protein, respectively. This balance between the three kinds of nutrients results in a more stable blood sugar level. A stable blood sugar level, in turn, helps you to control hunger and permits you to function optimally on less food (that is, fewer calories) than you would be likely to eat with a fluctuating blood sugar level.

To put it another way, the calories you derive from carbohydrates, fats, and proteins in the 40/30/30 food paradigm won't cause hunger pangs—even though you will be eating less food.

CHAPTER 2

IS THE 40/30/30 DIET RIGHT FOR YOU?

AS DESCRIBED EARLIER, THE 40/30/30 DIET IS A BALANCE OF 40 percent (slow-acting) complex carbohydrates that are fiber rich and mostly low glycemic; 30 percent lean, complete protein; and 30 percent quality fats.

That remarkable equation works equally well for both women and men. After all, dieting isn't just for women. The truth is that men throughout the country are more overweight than women are. Unfortunately, only about 47 percent of men are really concerned with their nutritional intake. However, a growing number are becoming more concerned about their appearance, even opting for cosmetic surgery. In fact, at the recent International Congress of Esthetics in Miami in October 2001, I learned that approximately 30 percent of cosmetic surgeries performed over the past twenty-five years were done on men.

Actually, more men need to get involved with good nutrition because male obesity typically centers around the middle of the body—a much more harmful obesity pattern than that found on women. This male pattern is related to various health risks: cardiovascular disease, diabetes, gallbladder disease, hypertension, musculoskeletal problems, sleep apnea, stroke, and even some cancers. But there's good news for men. For physiological reasons, they tend to drop those extra pounds a lot faster than women can.[1]

Whether male or female, however, everyone needs to adopt a sound nutritional approach for proper weight as well as for better health. One can actually increase longevity by losing weight. Just dropping 10 percent of one's weight can be a big help toward becoming a more vibrant and healthier person.

Is the 40/30/30 plan right for you? Find out by answering the following ten questions.

IS THE 40/30/30 PLAN RIGHT FOR YOU?

1. Have you failed to lose weight—or even gained some—while sticking to a low-fat, high-carbohydrate diet? Yes ❑ No ❑
According to some experts, in three out of four Americans an excess of processed carbohydrates and simple sugars in the diet cause an oversecretion of insulin into the bloodstream. This hormone helps in the buildup of fatty tissue.

2. Do you have midmorning or midafternoon drops in energy level? Yes ❑ No ❑
If you have energy "lows" a few hours after meals, you can be reasonably certain that you are eating too many processed carbohydrates or simple sugars. They give you an energy boost as the blood sugar derived from them is quickly used up—and then they leave you sagging with a low blood sugar level.

3. Do you have sugar cravings? Yes ❑ No ❑
These cravings occur when your blood sugar level falls too low. Eating something sweet brings the level back up—and reinforces your sugar habit. A combination of high-calorie, high-sugar snacks and fluctuating blood sugar levels is enough to sabotage most old-style weight-loss plans.

4. Do you often experience bloating or water retention?
Yes ❑ No ❑

Too much insulin secretion is frequently responsible for these symptoms and encourages the layering of body fat. Cutting back on processed carbohydrates and simple sugars as well as welcoming back unsaturated fats and protein into your diet can reduce weight due to both water retention and adipose tissue.

5. Do you have cravings for high-fat meat and dairy products?
Yes ❑ No ❑

If you do, you may burn carbohydrate calories more quickly than other people. People with a fast metabolism need dietary fats to slow down the consumption of calories and maintain a more balanced blood sugar level.

6. Do you exercise and still don't lose weight? Yes ❑ No ❑

When your body needs energy, it burns up all available carbo-hydrates first. So if you eat a high-carb diet, your body never needs to resort to burning stored fats for its energy needs. Unsaturated fats in your diet actually encourage the burning up of stored fat in your body. They do this by helping in the produc-tion of eicosanoids, hormonelike substances. This is why, ironi-cally, a very low-fat diet may add weight, rather than take it off.

7. Does exercise wipe you out? Yes ❑ No ❑

If you seem to take longer than others to recover from exercise, you may be eating too little protein and fat to support weight loss. Protein helps repair and rebuild muscle tissue after exer-cise. If you have muscle soreness for quite a while after exercis-ing, it's very likely that you are eating too little protein to produce the hormone glucagon in sufficient amounts to com-bat insulin. Glucagon helps your body consume stored fat. If you lose weight while eating too little protein, you may be using up muscle tissue instead of fat tissue. When you eat too few fats, you may not produce eicosanoids in sufficient quantity to burn body fat.

8. Do you hunger for carbs the more of them you eat? Yes ❑ No ❑

The more carbs carbohydrate addicts get, the more they want. Cravings for carbs result from problems involving insulin and blood sugar levels boosted by carbohydrates. Carb-eating binges are likely to follow, and this is one sure way to pile on body fat.

9. Do you have high cholesterol, high triglycerides, high blood pressure, or adult-onset diabetes? Yes ❑ No ❑
The presence of one or more of these risk factors for cardiovascular disease may indicate an underlying condition of insulin resistance. When the body becomes increasingly unresponsive to insulin, both blood sugar and insulin levels become high, with consequent weight gain and risk to health.

10. Are you an apple or a pear? Yes ❑ No ❑
People who put on weight around their abdomen (apples) tend to develop even more weight and health problems than people who put on weight on their hips and thighs (pears). If you carry excess abdominal fat, you should do well on the 40/30/30 diet.

HOW DID YOU SCORE?

Even if you answered yes to only one of these ten questions, the 40/30/30 diet may be just what you are looking for. In fact, most 40/30/30 advocates report dramatic weight loss and effortless weight maintenance (without hunger or feeling deprived) as well as level blood sugar values, no more cravings, and long-term energy.

Keep in mind that individual bodies vary greatly in their nutrient requirements. Not everybody, as I've said before, may need as much protein and fat as this eating program suggests. Individual variation in the 40/30/30 diet based upon ancestry, metabolism, and blood type is covered in Chapter 8. Because of biochemical individuality, it simply isn't possible to tailor a single dietary plan to fit everybody.

However, there is one suggestion that I think applies to everyone who has had trouble losing weight on the low-fat, high-carbohydrate regimen: Try out the basic 40/30/30 diet for size and let the results speak for themselves. And be sure to read on for a closer look at how the macronutrients—carbohydrates, fat, and protein—are viewed from a 40/30/30 perspective.

CHAPTER 3

CARBOHYDRATES FROM THE 40/30/30 PERSPECTIVE

THE CARBOHYDRATE COMPONENT (40 PERCENT OF TOTAL calories rather than the more typically recommended 55 to 70 percent) is the first macronutrient recommendation that flies in the face of the nutritional wisdom of the past two decades. I am devoting considerably more space to the carbohydrate section so that you will clearly understand why curtailing certain carbohydrates is essential to the success of the 40/30/30 concept. I will also introduce the glycemic index, which plays a major role in the choice of carbohydrates for consumption. The glycemic index, from the 40/30/30 perspective, is actually a much more important concept than the academic distinction between simple and complex carbohydrates. You will understand why as you read on.

As you may already know, carbohydrates, proteins, and fats are the three fundamental nutrients that our bodies absorb from food in our intestines. Of the three, carbohydrates are among the most efficient at supplying fuel for energy, in the form of glucose in our bloodstream. Carbohydrates may be simple or complex. Sugars are simple carbohydrates (often called simple sugars), consisting of only one or two units in each molecule such as sucrose (white sugar). Sugars are digested and absorbed quickly, supplying a quick source of energy.

Complex carbohydrates, in contrast, are built of chains of simple sugars. They are derived from starches such as grains, beans, and vegetables such as squash and potatoes. As a nutritionist, I was always taught that complex carbohydrates took longer than simple sugars to be digested and absorbed, thus entering the bloodstream more slowly for a longer-lasting and steadier source of energy.

Much to my surprise, I have since learned that certain complex carbohydrates such as potatoes, corn, and shredded wheat (the very ones we all have been loading up on for the past twenty years) are actually absorbed by our bodies quickly, in much the same way that simple sugars are.

THE GLYCEMIC INDEX

The glycemic index is a listing of carbohydrates that shows the rate at which a particular food breaks down as sugar or glucose into the bloodstream. Foods with a high glycemic index are considered to be fast acting because they release glucose into the bloodstream quickly, causing a rapid rise in blood sugar and then a rise in insulin, the fat-storage hormone par excellence. Foods with a low glycemic index are considered slow acting and release glucose into the bloodstream slowly but surely.

Arranging foods according to their glycemic index gives you a working knowledge of which foods to eat plentifully, moderately, and as little as possible. Certainly, foods assigned a high glycemic index are the most rapid inducers of insulin and, therefore, the ones to avoid.

Using the glycemic index allows you to offset one high-index food with several low-index foods. I highly recommend such "creative accounting." Even more importantly, the glycemic index (updated here based upon the latest research) can save you from the effects of unknowingly eating several high-index foods together.

Although the list of foods in the glycemic index may look a bit daunting at first, you will quickly catch on to the thinking behind it and be able to choose which foods work best for you. Accuracy of assigning percentage points is much less important than gaining an overall understanding of foods and insulin response. And you'll find this extensive index extremely helpful because it includes everyday name brands. Many of the foods are not always the most nutritionally desirable, but they are acceptable when combined with the right fats and proteins. Here are a few key points to keep in mind while reviewing the glycemic index.

GLYCEMIC INDEX POINTERS

Remember That . . .

- When processed carbohydrates are listed in the same category as whole grain products, they are still less beneficial because they lack the vitamins, minerals, and fiber that whole grain foods possess.

- When proteins and fats are eaten with high- or moderate-glycemic foods, they help slow down absorption of carbohydrates and therefore help prevent sharp rises in blood sugar and insulin levels.

- The kind of energy you feel is closely tied to this index. The higher the food is on the glycemic index, the faster the burst of energy and the sooner the letdown. Lower glycemic index foods provide a healthier, more long-term energy.

Much of the data in tables 3.1, 3.2, and 3.3 was obtained from *The Glucose Revolution: The Authoritative Guide to the Glycemic Index—The Groundbreaking Medical Discovery* by one of the world's leading authorities on the glycemic index, Jennie Brand-Miller, Ph.D., assisted by noted researcher Thomas M. S. Wolever, M.D., Ph.D., president of the Australian Diabetes Society; Stephen Colagiuri, M.D.; accredited dietitian-nutritionist Kay Foster-Powell, B.Sc.M.; and registered dietitian and certified diabetes educator Johanna Burani, M.S., R.D., C.D.E.[1]

TABLE 3.1. RAPID INDUCERS OF INSULIN

Glycemic index greater than 100 percent

Dried dates
Glucose powder
Maltose, pure
Tofu frozen dessert (nondairy)

Glycemic index between 90 and 99 percent

French baguette
Gluten-free spelt bread
Parsnips, boiled

Glycemic index between 80 and 89 percent

Corn Chex
Corn flakes
Grapenuts Flakes
Pretzels
Red-skinned potatoes, peeled
Rice cakes
Rice Chex
Rice, instant

Rice Krispies
Shredded wheat
Tapioca pudding
White potato, with skin, baked

Glycemic index between 70 and 79 percent

Bagel, small, plain
Bran flakes
Bread, rye
Bread, white
Cheerios
Corn chips
Gatorade sports drink
Graham crackers
Millet
Pumpkin
Raisin Bran
Rice, short grain, white
Rutabaga
Skittles fruit candy
Watermelon

TABLE 3.2.   MODERATE INDUCERS OF INSULIN

*Glycemic index
between 60 and 69 percent*

Beets
Bread, whole wheat
Cantaloupe
Cornmeal
Couscous
Croissant
Grapenuts
Hamburger bun
Ice cream, 10 percent fat, vanilla
Pineapple, fresh
Puffed Wheat
Raisins
Sucrose
Taco shells

*Glycemic index
between 50 and 59 percent*

Bread, pumpernickel,
   whole grain
Bread, sourdough
Corn
Peaches, canned
Pita bread, whole wheat
Popcorn, light

Rice, brown
Rice, long grain, white
Rice vermicelli, cooked
Semolina, cooked
Special K cereal
Sweet potato
Yam

*Glycemic index
between 40 and 49 percent*

Apple juice, unsweetened
Baked beans
Blackeyed peas
Bulgur, cooked
Chickpeas
Grapefruit juice, unsweetened
Grapes, green
Oatmeal, old-fashioned, cooked
Orange juice
Orange, navel
Pasta
Peach, fresh
Peas, green
Pineapple juice, unsweetened
Pinto beans
Rice, converted

TABLE 3.3. REDUCED INDUCERS OF INSULIN

Glycemic index
between 30 and 39 percent

Apple, raw
Apricots, dried
Beans, black
Beans, butter
Beans, mung
Beans, navy
Lentils, green and brown
Pear, fresh
Plums
Spaghetti, whole wheat
Yogurt, nonfat, fruit-flavored

Glycemic index
between 20 and 29 percent

Apples, dried

Barley, pearled, boiled
Cherries, fresh
Fructose
Grapefruit, raw
Lentils, red
Peas, dried

Glycemic index
between 10 and 19 percent

Agave nectar
Peanuts, roasted
Rice bran
Soybeans
Yogurt, nonfat, plain,
   unsweetened

INSULIN RESISTANCE

As the preceding tables show, simple sugars, processed carbohy-drates, and high-glycemic carbohydrates (such as rice cakes, cold cereals, and even whole wheat bread) when eaten alone are quickly digested in the intestines and absorbed by the body. That single act instigates a flood of glucose being released into the bloodstream, which triggers a blood sugar imbalance.

The pancreas secretes just enough insulin—a hormone needed to restore balance, supply fuel, and control chemical processes—to regu-late blood sugar levels. It does that by guiding digested food into cells, where their receptors allow the right amount of glucose to enter.

When functioning properly, this process defends vital organs such as the kidneys from being impaired by the ravages of excessive sugar, since it is toxic. The process does that by transporting glucose to muscles for energy consumption and to adipose tissue, where it is stored as body fat. Insulin also aids the metabolic conversion of glucose to glucagon, helping the central nervous system dispatch messages of when to eat or stop eating.

This remarkably efficient insulin system has evolved over thousands of years, responding to nutrients from natural, unprocessed foods. A landmark study on Paleolithic nutrition published in the *New England Journal of Medicine* in 1985 found that our Stone Age bodies were well equipped to readily digest natural, unprocessed carbohydrates in the form of high-fiber vegetables and fruits. [2]

Today, however, it's a whole new ballgame. Our bodies have to face tremendous challenges, thanks to our twenty-first-century diet lifestyle. The normal insulin process can't handle the excessively sugar-ridden, high-carb processed foods we consume, nor has it had sufficient time to adapt. And since it can't function the way it was designed to, the storage and use of both blood sugar and fat are hindered.

For quite some time now, nutritionists have been stressing the role of insulin and other hormones, since their link to good health is undeniable. Unfortunately, the nutritionists' warnings were often unheeded. Today we are on the brink of another epidemic that is spreading across the nation. It's called *insulin resistance*.

Hormone specialist Gerald Reaven, M.D., from the Stanford University School of Medicine, championed a series of revealing studies over the past thirty years. He uncovered critical data about how the body uses and responds to insulin, publishing the first paper on insulin resistance—which is at the core of a condition known as Syndrome X. [3] Previously found most predominantly in the elderly, this rising health concern is characterized by impaired glucose tolerance, elevated triglycerides, high blood pressure, and low "good" HDL cholesterol. It is now showing up in even the young, affecting 60 to 75 million Americans. Sufferers usually feel tired after meals and may notice blood pressure and blood fat levels steadily climbing with each passing year.

Insulin resistance occurs when cells alter and impede insulin entry. Invariably, that leads to an abundance of insulin remaining in the blood longer than it should. As mentioned earlier, insulin normally eases the movement of glucose. But when there are increasingly elevated insulin levels in the bloodstream, the availability of cell receptor sites is reduced, which renders the insulin virtually useless.

"The more sugar an individual consumes," according to author Dr. Gary Evans, "the less effective insulin becomes because the body cells have to protect themselves from being overcome by too much glucose."[4] The bottom line remains: the more carbs consumed—no matter what the source—the more insulin released. When insulin does its job effectively, it's quite good at moving glucose off into fat storage. But that creates a glucose shortage in the blood. The body gets the message to increase blood sugar . . . and we end up eating more carbs. Fatigue follows every time blood sugar drops, so the vicious cycle begins again, and we find ourselves overdosing on more and more carbs, simple or complex, because our blood sugar is constantly low.

The fact is that the older we get, the less we need carbs for energy. And years of consuming sugar-rich, high-carb foods produce such a buildup of chronic high sugar levels that cells can no longer accept any more sugar molecules. The pancreas then has to release more insulin to reduce the sugar overload, creating an excessive amount of insulin in the bloodstream. That causes more cell receptors to shut down, fueling insulin resistance even further.

The overabundance of sugar in the bloodstream produces glycation—a process whereby glucose molecules bind to proteins in the body and create a "browning effect," a phenomenon of aging. Since the cells can't properly respond to glucose, the tissues turn off their insulin recognition switch and redirect the glucose to fat cells in the liver. In 5 to 10 percent of insulin-resistant sufferers, the sugar simply stays in the bloodstream when the fat cells become filled, leading to type 2 diabetes.

LIVING DANGEROUSLY

Our obsession with sugary, highly processed foods takes its toll in even more ways. To begin with, the high-carb trend goes hand in hand with the attempt to maintain a low-fat (and typically low-protein) diet. The excessive intake of carbohydrates creates fertile ground for insulin resistance and protein and fat deficiency. Futhermore, carbohydrates, in contrast to proteins, can't build muscle. So when we rely on a high-carb diet plan, we can also expect reduced muscle mass down the line.

The consequences of chronic increased insulin levels produce numerous additional health risks. Since excess calories can transform into triglycerides and cholesterol, the potential for coronary heart disease escalates. According to Dr. Reaven, Syndrome X could be the "surest route to a heart attack" and an equally "powerful predictor of coronary heart disease as elevated cholesterol or LDL (bad) cholesterol, if not more so."[5] He found that Syndrome X sufferers are not only more likely to form blood clots but also are not as able to dissolve the blood clots, which dramatically raise the risk of heart attacks.

Accelerated aging can also be a potential risk factor. The more glucose in the system, the more it spontaneously oxidizes and releases even more free radicals. Linked to wrinkles, aging, and gray hair, free radicals negatively impact our looks and affect our well-being. Recent studies have shown that high sugar levels stimulate the production of free radicals, decrease vitamin E levels, and cause plaque buildup in arteries.[6]

Here's what happens. Excess sugar in the bloodstream becomes sticky like glue and clings to amino acid clusters in tissue proteins. These proteins then bind together (cross-link) into brownish substances called advanced glycosylation end products (AGEs). Biochemist Anthony Cerami discovered AGEs thirty years ago while studying the effects of sugar on the aging process, using diabetics as his model population group, since they tend to age more quickly.[7]

The glycosylation process transforms the integrity of proteins, which prevents them from performing properly. And which protein is the first to get hit? Collagen—a vital skin protein that gives skin its firmness and elasticity. It also is the connective tissue netting muscles to bone and keeping the entire skeleton intact. Collagen is instrumental in the lungs, cartilage, and blood vessels as well. When proteins go awry and AGEs are created, the skin's moisturizing agent decreases and collagen fibers turn flaccid, resulting in a thin epidermis, lines, and wrinkles.

The cold, hard truth is that the more AGEs we have, the faster we age. As Dr. Robert Atkins states, "hyperinsulinism [insulin resistance] accelerates aging . . . even small elevations in glucose and insulin levels affect your health as you age and are closely related to the chronic disorders of aging, including heart disease, cancer, and diabetes."[8]

Another health risk is hypoglycemia, which occurs when blood sugar levels are low. It's a frequent cause of fatigue, lack of concentration, mood swings, irritation, or anxiety and often precedes adult-onset diabetes. In many people its cause is nutritional—large secretions of insulin from the pancreas into the bloodstream in response to carbohydrate overload and ingested sugar eaten alone, as in desserts and soft drinks.

Without a doubt, consuming a sugar-filled, high–processed carb diet can destroy one's health in a number of ways. Here is a list of the most common disorders of the twenty-first century that are associated with unbalanced eating, particularly excessive intake of processed, high-glycemic carbohydrates:

- Acidic stomach
- Acne
- Adult-onset diabetes
- Alzheimer's disease
- Anxiety
- Appendicitis
- Asthma
- Atherosclerosis
- Blood clots
- Candidiasis
- Chromium deficiency
- Constipation
- Copper deficiency
- Coronary disease
- Crohn's disease
- Depression
- Drowsiness
- Early menopause

- Eating disorders
- Elevated blood pressure
- Excessive weight gain
- Fatigue
- Food allergies
- Gallbladder problems
- Gastrointestinal disorders
- Gastrointestinal problems
- Glucose intolerance
- Headaches
- High LDL cholesterol
- High triglyceride levels
- Hormone imbalance
- Hyperactivity
- Hypertension
- Immune compromise
- Impaired immunity
- Infertility

- Insomnia
- Irritable bowel syndrome
- Low HDL cholesterol
- Migraines
- Mineral imbalances
- Mood swings
- Osteoarthritis
- Osteoporosis
- Overstressed pancreas
- Periodontal problems
- Poor eyesight
- Serotonin production
- Stroke
- Tooth decay
- Varicose veins
- Various cancers
- Water retention

According to Dr. Reaven's 1995 study published in *Physiological Reviews*, the magnitude of the sugar-carb impact on our health explains today's epidemic proportions of type 2 diabetes, cardiovascular disease, and impaired immune disorders.[9]

A CLOSER LOOK:
CARBOHYDRATE-CONNECTED DISORDERS

Adult-Onset Diabetes

Predicted as the upcoming pandemic lifestyle disease, type 2 diabetes accounts for approximately 98 percent of all cases of diabetes. A study from the Centers for Disease Control (CDC) and Prevention showed that diabetes as a whole affects nearly 16 million Americans, and 85 percent of all diabetes sufferers are overweight or obese.[10]

In fact, diabetes rose so dramatically in the United States during 1999 that the government recognized it as proof that we are in the midst of a growing epidemic. According to the CDC, this increase in obesity crosses practically every demographic line, regardless of age, race, or educational background. The sad truth is that over 50 percent of Americans are overweight. It should come as no surprise, then, that the rate of diabetes increased 70 percent among individuals still in their thirties.

Further proof of the obesity–diabetes connection came with a September 1999 study conducted by the CDC. Its research revealed that diabetes jumped 33 percent in American adults between 1990 and 1998—just as obesity steadily climbed from 18 percent in 1998 to 19 percent in 1999. The CDC's senior epidemiologist, Ali H. Mokdad, Ph.D., stated in a letter published in *Diabetes Care* that "when we look at obesity and diabetes, the association is as strong as that between smoking and lung cancer . . . the driving force in the increase in diabetes is obesity."[11]

Diabetes develops when there is a shortage of insulin or when the insulin is no longer effective in getting blood sugar into the muscle cells. As a result, the body can't metabolize the glucose, getting less of it for energy, which only causes more blood sugar to be stored as fat. Nerve and muscle cells become lethargic in the process as they are robbed of their main energy source.

Besides the decreased energy and increased body weight, a host of related health complications follow. In spite of treatment for their diabetes, diabetics often develop heart disease, blindness, kidney failure, hemorrhages, impaired circulation, strokes, and blood circulation problems. Capillary walls weaken and vessels become clogged, which can result in ulcerations on the legs and feet—often causing amputation as the only solution. And with the dreadful disease impacting a rising number of midteens, its disastrous impact may not show up until sufferers are in their thirties or forties. In fact, the potential for heart disease increases dramatically, doubling for men and quadrupling for women. Diabetes is also the second most frequent cause of male impotence, only just behind cardiovascular disease.[12] Some doctors, however, believe diabetes is the most frequent cause.

Most importantly, nearly 85 percent of all diabetics are either overweight or obese.[13] The heavier a person becomes, the higher that person's chance is for developing diabetes. According to endocrinologist Frank Venicor at the CDC, a lack of exercise coupled with a high-calorie diet puts one at risk. So it should come as no surprise that the United States has one of the highest diabetic rates in the world. In the late 1970s, 45 percent of Americans fell into the overweight/obese category. By the early 1990s, that figure had risen to 55 percent, according to the CDC. And in that same time frame, the figures doubled for teens.[14]

Venicor also reports that the thirty-something crowd has higher obesity levels as well as lower physical activity. Perhaps that explains why this age group had a 70 percent hike in diabetes cases between 1990 and 1998, compared to the 33 percent increase experienced overall for that period. According to JoAnn Manson of Harvard Medical School, more than 80 percent of diabetes cases are linked to overweight/obesity issues. As a matter of fact, she says that "obesity is more closely linked to diabetes than any other health problem." An overweight American woman actually has twice the risk for developing diabetes as a woman of "optimal" weight.[15] And a *Lancet* report indicates that being physically inactive doesn't help—it actually ups the chances, even if an individual isn't overweight.[16]

A first-rate scientific study supports the warnings that eating processed grains such as white rice, pasta, bread, and cold cereals is just as bad as (if not worse than) eating a lot of sugar with adult-onset diabetes. In February 1997, Dr. Jorge Salmeron and Harvard colleagues published the results of a study that tracked the diets of 65,173 women, forty to sixty-five years old, for six years.[17]

The study, the results of which appeared in the *Journal of the American Medical Association*, found that women who ate a starchy diet that was low in fiber and who drank a lot of soda became diabetic two and a half times more often than women who ate a healthier diet.

The overwhelming message of the study was that women who ate a lot of sugar, pasta, white rice, and potatoes in order to cut down on fats in their food were harming more than helping themselves. Their diet of starchy foods (potatoes), processed carbohydrates (rice, pasta, and bread), and sugar (in soda) amounted to frequent surges in blood sugar followed by increasing amounts of insulin required to break down the blood sugar and resulting in insulin resistance. As many as one in four Americans are thought to suffer to some extent from insulin resistance. Yet other researchers (such as Dr. Richard Heller and Dr. Rachel Heller of Mt. Sinai Hospital in New York and Dr. Michael Eades of Boulder, Colorado) feel that the number may be as high as three out of four.[18]

Cardiovascular Disease

Heart disease is the leading cause of death in America, responsible for 953,120 deaths in 1997; another 159,791 deaths were caused by strokes. When undiagnosed and miscellaneous related causes are added to National Center for Health Statistics data, the number of Americans who die annually from cardiovascular disease can be rounded out to over a million.

Among the first to notice the connection between sugar and cardiovascular disease was British researcher Dr. John Yudkin, whose 1972 classic *Sweet and Dangerous* described many instances in which sugar was a greater threat to health than dietary fats.[19] Two of his examples were the Masai and Sumburu peoples of East Africa, who eat a high-fat diet of mostly milk and red meat but no sugar—and who have almost no heart disease.

In his 1975 book *The Saccharine Disease*, Dr. T. L. Cleave linked sugar and processed carbohydrates to cardiovascular disease, diabetes, and other illnesses.[20] He noted that these ailments were often almost nonexistent in various societies before the people started eating processed carbohydrates. About twenty years after people began eating processed carbohydrates, cardiovascular disease and diabetes began to occur with alarming frequency.

As discussed earlier, eating too many sugary foods, processed carbohydrates, or high-glycemic carbs such as rice cakes, cold cereals, or a plain baked potato leads to a sudden rise in blood sugar levels, which is answered by the pancreas with a secretion of insulin into the bloodstream. Large amounts of insulin in the bloodstream are associated with high blood pressure, obesity, low levels of "good" cholesterol, and high levels of triglycerides. The threat implicit in high triglycerides, while acknowledged privately by most physicians, is not publicized in a forceful way because it has not been demonstrated beyond a shadow of a doubt in medical research.

However, in two of his published prospective studies, Dr. Reaven discusses a study published in the *Journal of Clinical Endocrinology and Metabolism* of 147 people who were near fifty years old. He measured their insulin resistance, then checked them in five years. Of the third who were most insulin resistant, one out of seven had experienced a heart attack. Nobody in the third who were the least insulin resistant had had a heart attack.[21] And in other research published in *Metabolism*, 650 individuals were observed over a ten-year period. Of the fourth with high insulin levels, nearly 8 percent had heart attacks, compared to only 1 to 2 percent in the remaining groups.[22] Paralleling these findings, a Quebec cardiovascular study described in the *New England Journal of Medicine* showed that approximately 70 percent of its subjects having heart disease also had Syndrome X, along with many of the risk factors mentioned earlier.[23] Most importantly, the study discovered that every 30 percent rise in insulin produced a 70 percent higher risk for heart disease throughout a five-year interval.

A potential link, noted by researchers at Yale University and Rockefeller University, could exist between a high-carb diet and elevated levels of triglycerides, which are made of fat. Insulin-resistant individuals have more fat being released into their bloodstream, causing the liver to generate even more triglycerides. That's a disturbing fact, since triglyceride levels are considered a better and more precise indicator of potential heart attacks. Not surprisingly, Dr. Reaven's research showed that the common denominator among heart attack sufferers was elevated glucose and triglyceride levels.[24]

A continual increase of insulin stimulates blood clot formation, widening the opportunity for blockages, rigid vessels, and high blood pressure as well as sodium and water retention. And the more elevated the blood pressure, the greater the risk for a stroke—a top killer, right under heart disease and cancer. Numerous tests performed on over 1,600 subjects over eighty years old, according to a *Lancet* paper, revealed that reducing blood pressure did just as good a job preventing strokes in the elderly patients as it did in youthful individuals.[25]

Cancer

Although sugar and processed carbohydrates have not been identified as direct causes of cancer, they indirectly promote the disease by providing instant fuel—glucose—which enables uncontrolled cell growth. Without this abundant fuel supply, cells would not have the energy to proliferate wildly.

In 1931, Otto Warburg, Ph.D., a German Nobel laureate in medicine, found that cancer cells increased during an anaerobic glycolysis process. During the process, glucose with lactic acid energized cancerous cells and created a lactic acid buildup, resulting in fatigue.[26]

A study done with sixty-eight mice injected with a breast cancer strain produced some eye-opening results. Some were put on diets to promote hyperglycemia (high blood sugar), normal blood sugar, or hypoglycemia (low blood sugar). Just seventy days later, the research demonstrated that those with normal to low blood sugar had a substantially higher survival rate. Only eight of the twenty-four hyperglycemic mice survived, whereas sixteen of the twenty-four with normal blood sugar and nineteen of the twenty hypoglycemic mice made it.[27]

And a four-year study conducted in the Netherlands by the National Institute of Public Health and Environmental Protection bolsters those findings. Comparing 111 biliary tract cancer patients with 480 controls showed that the risk connected with sugar intake doubled.[28] Adding to that, research performed in twenty-one nations—spanning North America, Japan, and Europe—traced morbidity/mortality statistics and found sugar intake to be the most powerful factor contributing to breast cancer rates, especially in older women.[29]

Impaired Immunity

Simple sugars and processed carbohydrates are immunosuppressants. In these times of viral and bacterial epidemics, much increased international travel, and relaxed sexual mores, anything that suppresses our immune system has to be regarded as a grave threat to our health. Sugar and refined carbohydrates appear to suppress the immune system in the following five ways:

1. After ingestion, they destroy the germ-killing powers of white blood cells for as long as five hours.
2. They lessen the production of antibodies, which hone in on foreign invaders in the bloodstream.
3. They interfere with the transport of vitamin C, one of the body's most important nutrients and antioxidants.
4. They weaken the immune system by causing mineral imbalances and sometimes allergic reactions.
5. They make cells more permeable and therefore vulnerable to invaders by neutralizing the action of essential fatty acids.

40/30/30: THE RIGHT DIET FOR INSULIN AWARENESS

According to Dr. Reaven, various factors, such as possible gene anomalies, ethnicity, and family history, can lead to insulin resistance. However, the most significant step one can take to offset insulin resistance is a lifestyle change. In fact, 20 to 25 percent of developing insulin resistance is connected to weight gain, and another 20 to 25 percent is contingent upon physical fitness. Thus, an average person losing just ten to fifteen pounds could benefit greatly.

Although Americans have reduced their dietary intake of fats over the last decade, they have become more overweight during the same period. It's understandable that many erroneously believe that if a food has little or no fat, it will not add to our body fat. But the truth is that all excess blood sugar, not used for energy by our muscles, is stored as body fat—regardless of what kind of food it came from. Carbohydrates can therefore create a bigger weight problem than fats for obese people.

Looking at food as the most powerful and ubiquitous drug we have, many nutritionists say that we need to eat in a controlled fashion and in the proper proportions. High-carb diets are definitely not the answer, especially since we have to secrete more insulin to handle carbs. The key is the 40/30/30 plan, which limits carb intake to 40 percent of calories.

In addition to taking insulin and other hormones into account, the 40/30/30 phenomenon can be personalized one step further according to your blood type, ancestry, and oxidation rate. No other dietary approach incorporates all these factors. The good news for 40/30/30 followers is this: reducing all carbohydrates to 40 percent of total calories, being careful to select moderate-glycemic to low-glycemic choices, avoiding excessive refined carbohydrates, and lowering sugar consumption will cause that whole host of ailments to take care of itself.

The key is to remember that white rice may be even more dangerous than white sugar. According to Harvard researchers, eating processed carbohydrates, measured ounce for ounce, raises blood sugar levels more than eating pure sugar itself. Of course, that doesn't mean sugar is good for you. What it does suggest is that some processed carbohydrates are actually worse.

There are other things you can do to maintain a healthy blood sugar level. The next chapters will share some of these effective, simple tips.

CHAPTER 4

FATS FROM THE 40/30/30 PERSPECTIVE

AN IRRATIONAL FEAR OF FAT HAS BROUGHT WITH IT THE carbohydrate craze that is responsible for the burgeoning of the American waistline. While not all fats are good (particularly fried, oxidized, hydrogenated, or heat-processed fats, such as those in fried foods, margarine, and vegetable shortening), we can't overlook the fact that not all fats are bad. Moreover, some fats are even essential. The problem is that for the past fifteen years, most Americans have been eating an excess of the worst kind of fats.

Voices of reason (including mine) were raised during the widespread media demonization of *all* fats, but they were not often heard. Looking back now, it's hard to understand how so many supposedly knowledgeable diet experts could deny that our good health, and even our lives, depend upon our consuming quality and protective fats such as extra-virgin olive oil, flaxseed oil, fish oils, nuts, seeds, and avocado.

In terms of the 40/30/30 concept, fats are primarily important because they slow down the digestion of carbohydrates into the system, which helps keep insulin levels lower. Certain fats provide the essential fatty acids that become part of the eicosanoids—hormones we'll discuss in Chapter 6 that play a significant role in every phase of our daily health. In addition, as our most concentrated energy source (supplying 9 calories per gram), fats make food taste good and release the hormone cholecystokinin (CCK) from our stomach to send a message of satiety to our brain when we have eaten sufficiently. Without that message, we continue to feel hungry.

Plain and simple, our bodies couldn't function without fats. Perhaps this is why such prestigious organizations as the American Heart Association suggest that we should be consuming up to 30 percent of total calories from this essential nutrient. Researchers at the Harvard School of Public Health admit that "low-fat diets have only caused people to eat more sugar and more calories . . . there's good evidence that a moderate-fat diet would be healthier than a low-fat one."[1] Fats are required for hormone production, facilitation of oxygen transport, and calcium absorption as well as for the absorption of the fat-soluble, beautifying vitamins A, D, E (the premier antioxidant), and K—absolutely essential for radiant, youthful-looking skin and luster-rich hair.

Fats also help in:

- Preventing eczema; dandruff; psoriasis; dry skin, hair, and nails; and hair loss
- Slowing the aging process
- Protecting against osteoporosis, arthritis, heart disease, cancer, allergies, and asthma
- Lubricating cell membranes
- Helping cells function optimally so they can fight bacteria and viruses

Most importantly, fats make sure the detoxification process is running at its peak, seizing oil-soluble poisons lodged in fatty tissues and escorting them out for elimination.

Even muscles opt for fats over glucose because fats produce more energy, giving us another incentive to protect our insulin process.[2] If the insulin system malfunctions, fat can't be transported from either fat cells or muscle cells, and glucose is used as a backup choice. That, however, produces a loss of muscle mass. And in the interim, other cells fill the void and gradually transform into fat cells. Can you guess what happens after that? More weight gain.

THE REMARKABLE OMEGAS

Including good-for-you fats in your diet—those from the omega family—guarantees an array of health and weight-management benefits. These fats are necessary companions for weight control, since they produce long-term appetite satisfaction, which means you'll eat less and not be tempted to overindulge. Quite simply, the fats from the omega family regulate metabolic processes all the way down to the cellular level, helping the cardiovascular, immune, reproductive, and central nervous systems on a minute-to-minute basis each and every day.

The remarkable omegas also soothe skin, promote healing, and regulate water loss. Their anti-inflammatory properties help to dilate blood vessels for improved blood flow; help control blood clotting; and reduce the swelling, pain, and redness produced by bodily injuries. And since the good fats aren't stored by the body, we have to consume sufficient amounts of omega fatty acids daily to ensure their production.

The Omega-3s

Recent research indicates that omega-3s prevent blood clotting; repair tissue damage caused by clogged arteries; lower the rate at which the liver makes triglycerides; lower high blood pressure; and protect the body from autoimmune diseases, such as rheumatoid arthritis, in which the body is attacked by its own immune system.

Found in fatty fish, flaxseed, walnuts, pumpkin seeds, and even leafy greens, omega-3s have also been shown to retard yeast overgrowth in the body, which is often associated with various digestive and reproductive symptoms, and recurring bladder infections as well as acne and itchy, scaly rashes.

Some of the more interesting benefits of omega-3s occur when it converts to the acid known as docosahexaenoic acid (DHA). Studies indicate that DHA may thwart insulin resistance. Others reveal that low DHA levels tend to appear in obese individuals.[3] And DHA nourishes neurons and brain cells. In fact, Alzheimer's disease is linked to low DHA levels in the blood. Perhaps it's no wonder that omega-3 fatty acids greatly support such challenges as attention deficit hyperactivity disorder (ADHD). As a matter of fact, seven-time Nobel Prize nominee Dr. Johanna Budwig—who has spent over fifty years researching the healing benefits of fats—believes that "normalizing the fat intake in our nutrition would have a tremendous effect on social behavior."[4]

Numerous other studies of omega-3s, particularly in fish and flaxseed, demonstrate its impact on heart health, since the fatty acid helps reduce triglyceride levels. According to Neil J. Stone, M.D., using fish oil supplements "is an important therapeutic option" when treating high blood fat levels.[5] In fact, fish oil has been shown to retard production of LDL—the bad cholesterol, which can accumulate and restrict circulation. That may well have been a factor behind the findings of researchers who studied the Greenland Inuit population, whose diet centers on large amounts of fish and fish oil. The researchers found the death rate from heart disease to be lower than that in other nations.[6]

Medical researchers in Seattle, Washington, discovered that individuals whose diets included omega-3s suffered 50 percent fewer heart attacks than those whose diets did not.[7] And a report in the *American Journal of Cardiology* revealed that patients recuperating from heart bypass surgery had few problems with new blood vessels when fed omega-3s.[8]

Of great importance to women is the fact that omega-3-rich flaxseed contains potent antioxidant fiberlike substances known as lignans. The lignans in flax have the ability to stabilize blood sugar, keep appetite down, and balance estrogen metabolism, which helps reduce premenstrual symptoms. Their hormone-balancing properties also help the mature woman by decreasing postmenopausal hot flashes and vaginal dryness. Lignans may even have an impact on preventing osteoporosis. The most powerful benefit of lignans, however, may be in fighting breast cancer. In Perth, Western Australia, researchers conducted a 1997 *Lancet* study and discovered an amazing reduction in breast cancer risk among women who had a high intake of lignans like those in flaxseed oil.

The Omega-6s

If you really want to burn fat as well as be proactive against rheumatoid arthritis, diabetic neuropathy, eczema, and psoriasis, then you should also include the "good" omega-6 fatty acids such as gamma linolenic acid (GLA), found in borage oil, evening primrose oil, and black currant seed oil. These beneficial essential fatty acids (EFAs) have been shown to possess an uncanny ability to fire up metabolism, not to mention moisturizing flaky skin, dry hair, and brittle nails. The GLA in omega-6 oils helps with weight loss by stimulating brown fat metabolism—a special fat-burning tissue that disperses surplus calories for heat instead of for fat storage. The result? You lose weight.

The Promise of CLA

There is now ground-breaking research on the omega-6s in the dietary supplement conjugated linoleic acid (CLA). Exhaustively studied since its discovery over a decade ago, CLA has demonstrated an ability to help on many health fronts. Researchers from the University of Wisconsin believe that we are getting no CLA from the foods we eat today due to two major factors. The first factor is the no- to low-fat mindset that has prevailed over the past several decades and steered Americans away from the only possible CLA dietary sources available—beef, lamb, and whole-fat dairy products like cheese, milk, and butter. The second factor is that livestock is no longer grass fed, but instead is raised in feedlots on grains, which decrease livestock's levels of CLA by nearly 80 percent. Thus, even people who consume animal protein are missing out on this important nutrient.

Laboratory research over the past twenty years has shown that CLA reduces the body's ability to store fat for energy by controlling the enzymes that release fat from the cells into the bloodstream. Lack of this critical fatty acid in the American diet is definitely a contributing factor to the steady rise in obesity over the past thirty years, even though we have reduced our overall fat intake. The long-awaited results of a year-long U.S. clinical trial led by Dr. Richard Atkinson[9] the president of the American Obesity Association, were reported at a meeting of the American Chemical Society in August 2000.

Atkinson's study was designed to determine the effects of CLA on body composition in obese men and women. The results were impressive. In his clinical trial of eighty overweight people who dieted and then regained weight, it was discovered that those who took CLA put the pounds back on in a ratio of half fat to half muscle—an extraordinary result considering that most regained pounds are usually redeposited as 75 percent fat and 25 percent muscle.[10] Dr. Michael Pariza, director of the Food and Research Institute at the University of Wisconsin, has been conducting research on CLA and obesity since the discovery of CLA in 1978.[11] Today there are more than one hundred studies on this previously unrecognized nutrient.

As reported in *U.S. News and World Report*, the first human clinical trial was conducted by MedStat Research Ltd. of Lillustrom, Norway, in 1997.[12] The ninety-day double-blind trial on twenty humans demonstrated a stunning 20 percent decrease in body fat percentage with an average reduction of seven pounds of fat in the group taking CLA versus no change in the placebo group. The subjects experienced very little change in body weight, which means their lean muscle mass increased proportionately to their decrease in body fat. So if you lose total body fat to the tune of 20 percent of your body fat, but the scale doesn't budge that much, then you have gained muscle, which, pound for pound, weighs more than fat.

A study performed by the Department of Public Health and Caring Sciences, described in *Clinical Nutrition Research*, showed that CLA substitutes muscle for fat.[13] And according to Utah State University doctors, CLA saturates the muscle cells and stimulates a 5 percent increase in metabolism. In other words, CLA works by reducing the body's ability to store fat and promotes the use of stored fat for energy. The result is a decrease in body fat and a proportional increase in lean muscle mass. The bottom line is this: Pound for pound, muscle burns more calories than fat, and every pound of muscle gained will burn seventy calories per hour without you even lifting a finger!

CLA may even help with adult-onset diabetes, according to a study headed by researcher Martha Belury, Ph.D., at Purdue University in Indiana. In the eighty-eight-week study, 64 percent of the twenty-two participants who took CLA demonstrated improved insulin levels.[14] Researchers at the Roswell Park Cancer Institute in Buffalo, New York, say CLA may be an extremely potent anticancer agent. According to cancer research scientist Dr. Clement Ip, CLA lowers the occurrences and number of mammary tumors. Dr. Ip conducted a study that gave high doses of carcinogens to rats, then fed them either CLA-fortified butter or a regular diet having much lower CLA levels. Approximately 50 percent of the CLA subjects had breast tumors, a much lower rate than the 93 percent of the regular diet group that developed cancer.[15] Since CLA is stored in fat cells, it is thought that breast tissue—which is primarily fatty—is receiving a sustained amount of CLA.

Other researchers are suggesting that people can reduce LDL cholesterol by ten points in twelve weeks and reduce triglycerides 50 percent by taking 3,000 milligrams of CLA each day.[16]

The Omega-9s

Although omega-9s aren't essential, they are necessary for promoting good health. A monounsaturated fatty acid called oleic acid tops the omega-9 list of oils. Olive oil is perhaps the best oleic acid source; however, avocados, peanuts, almonds, pistachios, pecans, cashews, hazelnuts, and macadamias are also rich in oleic acid. And these fatty acids boast a high satiety factor, which reduces overeating.

A study done at the University of Milan in Italy demonstrated that omega-9s can actually guard arteries from plaque.[17] Additional research, headed by Dr. Scott Grundy at the University of Texas Health Science Department, on the coronary health benefits of omega-9 monounsaturated oils revealed some intriguing findings. Grundy reported in *The New England Journal of Medicine* that the monounsaturated type of fatty acid (oleic acid) in olive oil proved more beneficial at protecting arteries from cholesterol buildup than popular low-fat/high-carbohydrate diets.[18]

A well-known study of over 26,000 Seventh-Day Adventists confirmed that eating omega-9-rich nuts five times per week could help cut the chance of heart attack in half. The research, published in the *Archives of Internal Medicine* in 1992, cited the monounsaturated fat in the nuts as the prime catalyst for the heart disease decrease.[19]

Omega-9s also have been linked to breast cancer prevention. Dr. Alicja Wolk conducted a study in Stockholm that showed that women with the lowest intake of monounsaturated fats actually had the highest risk of breast cancer. According to Dr. Wolk, "It is a question of replacing one fat with another."[20] The point is to substitute trans-fats and saturated fats with healthy omega-3, omega-6, and omega-9 oils.

Even more importantly, the effects of omega-3 fatty acids can be enhanced by the oleic acid in omega-9 monounsaturated oils, which strengthens cell function and increases fluidity of the cell structure.

MAJOR FOOD SOURCES OF FATS

Both dietary and body fats are composed of a combination of one to three fatty acids and a molecule of glycerol, an alcohol. Fats are known as monoglycerides, diglycerides, or triglycerides, depending on their number of fatty acids. Fatty acids are the building blocks of fats, and at least two of them—linoleic and alpha-linolenic acid—are not made by the body and have to be obtained from food.

The structure of the fat molecule determines whether a fat is saturated or unsaturated. Saturated fats have all possible hydrogen atoms present. Unsaturated fats do not and are called monounsaturated or polyunsaturated, depending on whether they have one or more double bonds between adjacent carbon atoms. A simple way to tell the difference between them is that at room temperature saturated fats are solid and unsaturated fats are liquid. Another thing to keep in mind is that, contrary to what many people think, unsaturated fats do not, as a general rule, have fewer calories than saturated fats. Most fats are a mixture of saturated, polyunsaturated, and monounsaturated, with one kind predominating. And when eaten in moderation and in balance with the essential fatty acids, saturated fats are not as harmful or dangerous as most people believe.

	At Room Temperature	*Refrigerated*
Saturated fats (except tropical oils)	Solid	Solid
Polyunsaturated fats	Liquid	Liquid (except when hydrogenated)
Monounsaturated fats	Liquid	Semisolid or solid

The following paragraphs describe the major food sources for each fat group.

Saturated Fat

Animal sources: pork; lamb; beef fats (lard, tallow, suet); organ meats; full-fat dairy products such as whole milk, cream cheese, ice cream, butter

Vegetable sources: coconut oil, cocoa butter, palm oil, palm kernel oil

Monounsaturated Fat

Vegetable, legume, and seed sources: olives, avocados, almonds, apricot kernels, peanuts, high-oleic safflower and sunflower oils

Polyunsaturated Fats (Omega-3s)

Animal sources: salmon, mackerel, herring, cod, sardines, rainbow trout, shrimp, oysters, halibut, albacore tuna, sable fish, bass, flounder, anchovies

Vegetable sources: flaxseed oil, pumpkin seed oil, soybeans, walnuts, wheat germ, wheat sprouts, fresh sea vegetables, leafy greens

Polyunsaturated Fats (Omega-6s)

Animal sources: mother's milk, organ meats, lean meats

Vegetable sources: safflower, sunflower, corn, soy, sesame oils; raw nuts and seeds; legumes; spirulina; leafy greens

Botanicals: borage, evening primrose, and black currant seed oils

The Truth About Saturated Fats

Most people believe that saturated fats are the "bad fats" in our diet because they have been connected with high cholesterol and hardening of the arteries. This notion, however, is not only simplistic but it is incorrect.

Dr. Mary Enig, a well-respected researcher in the field of fats and oils, has demonstrated this repeatedly throughout her lifelong work. As far back as 1994, she stated in an eye-opening interview with biochemist Richard Passwater, Ph.D., that "the idea that saturated fats cause heart disease is completely wrong. However, the statement has been 'published' so many times over the last three or more decades that it is very difficult to convince people otherwise, unless they are willing to take the time to read and learn what all the economic and political factors are that produced the anti-saturated fat agenda in the first place."[21]

Several studies have shown that there is no increase in heart disease in countries or communities where most of the fat is either coconut oil or palm oil. Palm oil that is not extensively refined has very high levels of antioxidants, and coconut oil has high levels of very useful medium-chain fatty acids.

Understandably, you may be surprised by that last statement, since we've heard so much for so long about how bad palm oil and coconut oil are for us. But the truth is that although these tropical oils are high in saturated fat, they provide vital protective nutrients. In addition, coconut oil is considered one of the most stable oils and is therefore a viable alternative for both cooking and baking. Coconut oil also is important in the diet because nearly half of its fatty acid content is made up of an antiviral fatty acid known as lauric acid. For this reason, coconut oil may be the oil of choice for those individuals who are immunosuppressed. Palm oil has the most concentrated source of tocotrienols, a nutrient that's part of the vitamin E family. Tocotrienols can help lower cholesterol, prohibit clot formation, reverse atherosclerotic plaques, and hinder the spread of cancer cells.

In her book *Know Your Fats: The Complete Primer for Understanding the Nutrition of Fats, Oils, and Cholesterol*, Dr. Enig offers outstanding research that tells the true tale of how important fats are and which ones actually cause problems. She zeros in on the real culprits—partially hydrogenated vegetable fats and oils, with their trans-fatty acid troublemakers—and cites them as the catalysts behind many of our health problems. "Because trans-fatty acids disrupt cellular function," she writes, "they affect many enzymes . . . and consequently interfere with the necessary conversions of both the omega-6 and the omega-3 essential fatty acids to their elongated forms and consequently escalate the adverse effects of essential fatty acid deficiency."[22] According to Dr. Enig, our consumption of trans-fatty acids produces various adverse effects on both humans and animals. Consuming trans fats does the following:

- Lowers "good" HDL cholesterol
- Raises "bad" LDL cholesterol
- Raises the atherogenic lipoprotein in humans (while saturated fats lower it)
- Raises total serum cholesterol levels 20 to 30 percent
- Lowers the milk volume in lactating females in all species, including humans
- Decreases visual acuity in infants (up to fourteen months old)
- Correlates to low birth weight in humans
- Increases blood insulin levels in response to glucose load, upping the risk for diabetes
- Affects immune system response by lowering efficiency of B-cell response and increasing proliferation of T cells
- Decreases testosterone levels in male animals, decreases sperm levels, and interferes with gestation in females
- Decreases the response of red blood cells to insulin, causing a potentially undesirable effect in diabetes
- Inhibits the function of membrane-related enzymes
- Causes adverse alterations in vital enzyme system activities that metabolize chemical carcinogens and drug medications
- Alters physiological properties of biological membranes, such as membrane fluidity
- Alters adipose cell size, cell number, lipid class, and fatty acid composition

- Interacts adversely with conversion of plant omega-3 fatty acids to elongated omega-3 fatty acids
- Escalates adverse effects of essential fatty acid deficiency
- Potentiates free radical formation
- Precipitates childhood asthma

As you can see, the real villains causing our health problems may very well be vegetable fats in the form of processed vegetable oils, margarine, vegetable shortenings, and baked goods made from these products. A study conducted by Dr. Enig found that the use of animal fat has markedly decreased in the American diet for the past eighty years, falling from 83 to 53 percent of total fat intake. Conversely, there has been an enormous rise in vegetable fat intake, from 17 percent in 1910 to 47 percent in 1990. Enig has correlated the rise in vegetable fat consumption with the rise in cancer. Enig is especially concerned about vegetable fat in the form of the unnatural trans fats from hydrogenated and partially hydrogenated oil.

Foods highest in trans fats are the commercially made baked goods such as bread, crackers, rolls, muffins, biscuits, cookies, cakes, pies, and doughnuts. When McDonald's switched from beef tallow to partially hydrogenated vegetable oil for frying in 1990, the percentage of fat that came from trans-fatty acids in McDonald's french fries increased from 5 percent to between 42 and 48 percent. Trans fats are now believed to be connected not only to cancer, heart disease, and aging, but also to immune system suppression and diminished ability to utilize essential fatty acids.

Now that we've established how important fats are in the 40/30/30 concept, let's go on to the last vital macronutrient: protein.

CHAPTER 5

PROTEINS FROM THE 40/30/30 PERSPECTIVE

PROTEIN IS AN ESSENTIAL COMPONENT IN THE 40/30/30 program for several reasons. The first is that like dietary fat, protein has a stabilizing effect on blood sugar, thereby guaranteeing long-term, steady energy. Second, protein is important in the 40/30/30 plan because one of its most specific functions is to stimulate the production of the pancreatic hormone glucagon. Its role is opposite that of insulin. Glucagon helps to mobilize stored fat for use as a fuel source. So by eating lean, complete protein (such as eggs, fish, poultry, lean meat, low-fat cottage cheese, whey, and moderate soy), we lose weight by burning body fat for energy.

Vegetarians following the 40/30/30 plan can make their prime protein source eggs, low-fat cottage cheese, vegetable-based protein powders, and whey. Other sources of vegetable-based proteins such as beans and legumes, however, also contain substantial amounts of carbohydrate. Thus, too many beans and legumes may offset the proper nutrient balance of protein and carbohydrate.

While both carbohydrates and fats are involved in the energy process, proteins have an entirely different function. In the form of their building blocks—amino acids—they are used to maintain and repair muscles, body organs, blood, connective tissue, and skin. Protein is composed of twenty-two different types of amino acids. Nine of these are considered essential and must be supplied by the diet because the body cannot manufacture them on its own. We need a lot of protein to develop as infants and children. The manufacture of hormones and enzymes, healing of wounds, growth of hair and nails, and countless other biological processes are dependent on protein. The antibodies in our immune systems are protein. Nutrients and minerals are transported into and out of cells by amino acids. Because proteins are too large to pass through the walls of blood vessels, they can create osmotic pressure, drawing water toward them and thereby maintaining the water balance of the body.

Proteins provide four calories per gram. They can even be burned for energy, but this is not the most desirable or most effective way to generate energy. Except for pure fat and simple sugars, all foods contain some protein, but it is the complete proteins with high biological value (eggs, for example) that provide all of the essential amino acids.

As a primary food source, protein provides beautifying nutrients for lustrous hair, skin, and nails—all of which are 98 percent protein. Thus, consuming the proper amount of protein helps ward off droopy skin, dull hair, poor muscle tone, wrinkles, and sagging breasts.

Protein also plays a key part in the body's detoxification process, supporting the liver by escorting toxins and heavy metals out of the body. This is an essential function, since twenty-first-century life is burdened with potentially damaging metals, such as excess copper from copper water pipes, cookware, the Pill (estrogen retains copper), and some multivitamins, as well as copper-rich chocolate, tea, and soy. When protein is restricted, a copper overload occurs, creating numerous nutrient deficiencies such as zinc and vitamin C. Losing zinc robs us of an important mineral, needed to strengthen nails and hair, maintain unblemished skin, heal wounds and bruises, and keep menses regular.

Protein also helps with the production of a powerful antioxidant known as glutathione. This incredible nutrient stands on the fore-front, battling against disease, cancer, toxins, and aging. In fact, it has earned the name "the toxic waste neutralizer," since it is a major player in the detoxification process and fights toxic oxygen radicals.

Protein is an essential nutrient, which means the body can't store it. We must obtain the proper amounts daily. If we don't, our desire for carbohydrates (such as sugar) will gain the upper hand, with all its attendant problems.

CHAPTER 6

A TALE OF THREE HORMONES: INSULIN, GLUCAGON, AND THE EICOSANOIDS

THE 40/30/30 PHENOMENON IS BASED ON THE FACT THAT eating food evokes a hormonal response. As noted earlier, carbohydrates stimulate secretion of the hormone insulin. For simplicity's sake, it is important to remember that protein produces the hormone glucagon, and certain fats provide the building blocks of the tissuelike hormones known as eicosanoids. A more comprehensive biochemical approach would emphasize that a more important trigger for either insulin or glucagon is the level of sugar in the blood: low blood sugar triggers the pancreas to secrete glucagon, which in turn releases glycogen stores from the liver and fat energy from adipose tissue.

It is the delicate balance of carbohydrate, protein, and fat that determines the levels of these hormones in the body. Research has shown that the 40/30/30 proportion of these nutrients is the right eating equation to help most individuals stabilize blood sugar levels and lower fat-promoting insulin. In this way the body becomes a fat-burning machine without feelings of deprivation or hunger.

INSULIN

Insulin is the key hormone that controls blood sugar levels after one eats carbohydrates. Insulin helps muscle tissue use blood sugar as fuel for energy, and it helps store excess blood sugar in two ways. First, insulin helps store blood sugar in the liver and tissues as glycogen (a sugar). However, the body can store only a limited amount of glycogen. Any excess beyond what the body can store is converted to body fat, again with the assistance of insulin. To increase glucagon relative to insulin, and thus enable the body to access body fat better, requires a more balanced proportion of carbohydrate, protein, and fat at each meal. Along with a more balanced diet, exercise also reduces insulin levels.

Keep in mind that all the carbohydrates that our bodies absorb from food are converted into blood sugar, even from the least sugary of foods. But carbohydrates from low-glycemic food sources are converted more slowly into blood sugar, thus avoiding a rush of blood sugar and an answering rush of insulin into the bloodstream. Higher-glycemic carbohydrates (rice cakes and a baguette, for example) as well as simple sugars and processed carbohydrates (white rice and bagels, for example) produce these blood sugar and insulin rushes, with the consequent depletion of blood sugar, loss of energy and concentration, and renewal of food cravings.

GLUCAGON

The protein hormone glucagon works in opposition to insulin. What insulin puts away in storage, glucagon puts back into use. The two hormones do not conflict with one another in the bloodstream, because when the insulin level is high, the glucagon level is low and vice versa. When glucagon rises in the bloodstream, it is comparable to spending, not putting away. When you want to lose weight, this is the kind of "spending" you need to do.

When your blood sugar level drops, the pancreas secretes glucagon. It is believed that both protein-rich foods and exercise induce this process. Glucagon causes the stored sugar glycogen to be released back into the bloodstream to restore the blood sugar level. In addition to releasing glycogen, glucagon releases fat from adipose tissue. This fat is then burned as fuel and is thus lost by you, hopefully forever!

The different roles of insulin and glucagon can be summed up as follows:

Insulin	*Glucagon*
Lowers blood sugar level	Raises blood sugar level
Stores fat	Mobilizes fat from storage
Triggered by carbohydrates	Triggered by proteins

EICOSANOIDS

We need fats in our diet to provide the essential fatty acids that become part of the eicosanoids. Eicosanoids are natural hormones; that is, they are substances secreted by the body that have control over bodily functions. They are unusual in that they have very short lifetimes, existing for less than a few seconds. This short span of existence has made the study of eicosanoids difficult, and comparatively little is known about them. Prostaglandins are the only eicosanoids most people have heard of, and that is due to the importance of prostaglandins in the male sexual system. But eicosanoids have a much larger role to play in human biology than they are generally credited with. In fact, some authorities claim that eicosanoids control just about all hormones and every bodily function. They are known to be affected by the nutrients we absorb from food.

Like the different kinds of cholesterol, eicosanoids can be divided into "good" and "bad" categories. I place these words in quotation marks because neither category of eicosanoids is either good or bad in itself. Our bodies need both categories to be healthy. The most important thing is that both categories should be in—you guessed it—a state of balance.

From a nutritional point of view, the bad eicosanoids are so called because they tend to increase on a high-carbohydrate diet, with undesirable results in our bodies. Some physical results of good and bad eicosanoids are contrasted in the following lists.

Series 1 ("Good") Eicosanoids	Series 2 ("Bad") Eicosanoids
Dilate blood vessels	Constrict blood vessels
Retard blood clotting	Cause blood clotting
Dilate bronchioles	Constrict bronchioles
Retard cell proliferation	Increase cell proliferation
Strengthen immunity	Weaken immunity
Anti-inflammatory	Inflammatory
Lower cholesterol	Increase cholesterol
Decrease pain	Increase pain
Antidepressive	—
Stimulate endocrine hormones	—
—	Increase triglycerides

The insulin-glucagon balance in our bloodstream is also important, since too much insulin produces too many bad eicosanoids. Now, if this is beginning to sound too complicated, don't despair. All you really need to know is that when you eat according to the 40/30/30 principles, your body will be able to burn its own body fat for energy and, in so doing, give you more long-term appetite satisfaction and endurance on fewer calories.

In addition to taking insulin, glucagon, and the eicosanoids into account, the 40/30/30 phenomenon can be personalized further according to your ancestry, blood type, and metabolic rate. No other dietary approach incorporates these factors. Chapter 8 will tell you how.

CHAPTER 7

THE MINERAL FACTOR

THE BEST-KEPT SECRET IN NUTRITION HAS BEEN KEPT under wraps for nearly sixty-five years. And here it is: Minerals are the spark of life and even more important than vitamins. The U.S. government knew that back in 1936 when it issued a document stating, "Our physical well being is more directly dependent upon the minerals we take into our systems than upon calories or vitamins, or upon the precise proportion of starch, protein, or carbohydrate we consume."[1] So, as you continue to read this chapter, be thinking of how you can feature the most mineral-rich food sources in your 40/30/30 menu planning.

Many of us are aware that we can live for a prolonged period of time without food but not without water. One reason for this is because water provides our bodies with life-sustaining minerals. It works something like this: Every cell relies upon minerals for numerous bodily functions. And there are over seventy trillion cells in the human body, each one acting like a biological battery—a kind of minidynamo that generates life. Minerals are the catalysts to keep the battery going and help it hold a charge. Without minerals in the proper ratio, cellular membranes can't maintain the proper liquid pressure between the inside and outside cell walls. The imbalance causes cells to weaken and eventually die. Even the immune system depends upon this mineral-balancing act, right down to the cellular level.

As you know, no car can start without a well-running battery. The minerals of life recharge us on a minute-by-minute, daily basis, empowering every cell, organ, and tissue of the body.

WHAT CAN MINERALS DO FOR YOU?

Minerals do a lot. Besides their role in promoting blood formation, fluid regulation, protein metabolism, and energy production, minerals are also cofactors for enzyme catalysts for every biochemical response in the body. Minerals also maintain strong bones and teeth, help provide organ and glandular strength, and help relieve stress. However, since minerals are obtained through the soil, recognizing their value is one thing—getting them into your system is another matter altogether.

WHERE HAVE ALL THE MINERALS GONE?

Erosion breaks down rocks and stones containing mineral salts, causing them to become part of the soil that feeds plants. The minerals help plants bear fruit and grow. We get the minerals by eating either the plant's fruit or the animals that fed on the plant. Then, as plants die, the minerals return to the earth and feed other plants to keep the amazing cycle going.

That, however, is in a perfect world. In the real world, farmers strip plants and their fruit with the harvest, disrupting the vital circle of life and depleting the mineral content in the soil. Back when subsistence farming was more commonly practiced, people took only what they needed from the soil, so mineral reduction did not occur until hundreds or even thousands of years later. But the shift from rural to city living (over 85 percent of us now live in cities or their suburbs) forced the removal of plants and the depletion of valuable minerals.

Making matters worse, we've discarded the more traditional methods of organic farming, which relies upon crop rotation and manure fertilizers. Instead, most farmers use chemical fertilizer, such as NPK, which includes the elements nitrogen, phosphorus, and potassium. The potassium chloride used adds literally tons of chloride to each ton of potassium, which hinders a plant's ability to absorb magnesium and selenium. The chloride also leaches the soil of calcium and zinc. The nitrogen in NPK robs plants of iron and vitamin C as well. Farmers do attempt to put back some of the lost nutrients, but they depend upon the Department of Agriculture to tell them if it is needed. The Department of Agriculture's criteria, unfortunately, are based upon productivity levels, plant appearance, and plant growth. The nutritional value is not factored into the decision-making process.

Consequently, our plant production is up, and our plants look fine, but they are dangerously lacking in proper nutritional value. For instance, the calcium content of most leafy greens decreased by nearly 46 percent in the last generation; collard greens, however, lost 85 percent of their calcium content.[2] And the nutritional void also affects plant health, producing a rise in fungus, mold, and insect invasion. The modern-day solution to that problem is pesticides. The result? We have a high yield of good-looking, mineral-poor plants—loaded with poison. Understandably, our good health depends upon mineral supplementation.

KEY MINERALS

There are two groups of minerals: major (macro) and trace (micro). The macro are calcium, magnesium, phosphorus, potassium, sodium, and sulfur. The micro are chromium, copper, iodine, iron, manganese, selenium, zinc, and vanadium. Trace minerals—such as copper, boron, iodine, manganese, and chromium—are equally important because they allow the body to use proteins. As a matter of fact, most of us are deficient in the trace minerals required for electrolyte formation and homeostasis, which means we're absorbing only a small percentage of our protein intake. It also means we may have an upset in our pH balance and impaired digestion, hindering our ability to produce enzymes intended to metabolize protein and other nutrients. The rest of this chapter describes various minerals.

Macro Minerals

Calcium
Critical for bone building, teeth, and healthy gums as well as muscle growth. It helps lower cholesterol and guards against blood clotting.

Food sources: dairy, leafy greens, sea vegetables, salmon and sardines with bones, seafood, almonds, asparagus, blackstrap molasses, soybeans, oats, prunes, sesame seeds, tofu

Magnesium
Widely considered the most important mineral, it is involved in over 350 biochemical processes such as muscle contraction; nerve conduction; and preventing anxiety, irritability, asthma, and panic attacks. Major minerals (such as calcium, potassium, and sodium) are dependent upon its presence in order to function. Research conducted by one of the most distinguished magnesium experts in the United States, Dr. Mildred Seelig, suggests that a one-to-one ratio of both calcium and magnesium is essential for bones, teeth, and the prevention of hypertension and hardening of the arteries.[3] Other researchers support a two-to-one ratio in favor of magnesium. Magnesium gives your bones the flexibility and strength of ivory, which is a combination of about 50 percent magnesium and 50 percent calcium.

Food sources: green leafy vegetables, fish, meat, seafood, seeds and nuts (such as almonds), apples, apricots, avocados, bananas, blackstrap molasses, brown rice, cantaloupe, garlic, grapefruit, peaches, black-eyed peas, sesame seeds, soybeans, tofu, whole grains

Phosphorus

Phosphorus, along with its coworkers magnesium and potassium, helps to protect skin, bone, and teeth. It also helps to calm the nerves and heighten mental acuity.

Food sources: red meats, sardines, wheat germ, pumpkin seeds, almonds

Potassium

Regarded as a tremendous alkalizer, this mineral is critical to pH and water balance and is a natural diuretic. It has demonstrated an outstanding effect on keeping blood pressure low and is helpful in maintaining healthy, regular heartbeats. Potassium also aids the nervous system and supports adrenal gland functions, which is especially important because of today's stressful lifestyle. Research has suggested that potassium may help counteract tumor growth.

Food sources: dairy, fish, fruit (apricots, figs, bananas, raisins), legumes, meat, poultry, vegetables (potatoes, squash, yams), whole grains

Sodium

Natural sodium is of critical importance in neutralizing acidity and is necessary for hydrochloric acid production in the stomach. Sodium keeps arteries and veins pliable, and, due to its influence on calcium, it can help to dissolve stones in the kidneys, bladder, and gallbladder. Sodium also normalizes blood pressure and heartbeat and feeds the adrenals.

Food sources: sea salt, celery, carrots, beets, spinach

Sulfur

Sulfur is found in the highest concentrations in cartilage, tendons, and keratin, which is the tough protein substance found in hair and nails. No wonder sulfur is known as the "beauty mineral." Sulfur also is a potent detoxifier and helps the liver to dispose of waste products and toxins. It is involved in the production of hormones, antibodies, and enzymes.

Food sources: eggs, broccoli, cabbage, garlic, onions, green peppers

Trace Minerals

Chromium

Essential to glucose metabolism and energy, chromium is known as a fat burner. It helps to keep blood sugar levels stable and can protect against full-blown diabetes. Chromium also helps in the synthesis of cholesterol, fats, and proteins and can aid in attaining lean muscle mass.

Food sources: brewer's yeast, beer, brown rice, meat, cheese, whole grains

Copper

A double-edged sword, copper helps guard against heart disease and unsteady heart rhythms. A copper deficiency can raise cholesterol and blood pressure. Too much copper, however, creates a toxicity that can result in panic attacks and even yeast infections. Women should use copper-free multiple vitamins because excess copper— prevalent in the twenty-first-century lifestyle—is linked to estrogen dominance, an increasingly common condition synonymous with hormonal dysfunction.

Food sources: soy products, regular tea, cocoa, nuts, peas, beans, beets, avocados, radishes, lentils, liver, mushrooms, oranges, pecans, raisins, leafy greens, salmon, oysters

Iodine

Iodine aids in metabolizing excess fat. It also is vital for mental and physical development as well as thyroid gland functions. A deficiency has been related to fatigue, weight gain, and even breast cancer. However, an abundance could result in mouth sores, diarrhea, vomiting, and swollen salivary glands.

Food sources: iodized salt, sea salt, seafood, saltwater fish, kelp, lima beans, garlic, mushrooms, sesame seeds, soybeans, spinach, summer squash, chard, turnip greens

Iron

Needed for the oxygenation of red blood cells and hemoglobin production, iron helps support the immune system and is required for various enzymes. A deficiency can result in anemia, dizziness, digestive and swallowing problems, nervousness, obesity, brittle hair, frail bones, and hair loss, among other symptoms. However, studies have linked iron excess to escalated free radical production, heart disease, and cancer. Adult men and menopausal women should opt for iron-free supplements since these people may be more likely to have an iron buildup.

Food sources: red meat, dark green leafy vegetables, beans, beets

Manganese

A vital nutrient needed for fat, protein, and bone metabolism as well as enzymatic actions, manganese also helps bolster mental activities and faculties, ensuring strong nerves. Without it, vibrant health is simply not possible. A manganese deficiency could produce atherosclerosis, confusion, eye and hearing problems, elevated cholesterol levels, memory loss, hypertension, irritability, and other problems.

Food sources: avocados, nuts, seeds, whole grains, blueberries, egg yolks, dried peas, pineapples, leafy greens, legumes

Selenium

Selenium is a powerful antioxidant that bonds with unstable molecules, causing some researchers to feel that it inhibits cellular damage, premature aging, and potential cancer. Cornell University conducted a study using a daily supplement of 200 micrograms and discovered it caused a 50 percent reduction rate in cancer.[4] Scientists think the selenium-rich soil in Norfolk, England, may be one reason that residents there live longer than other English citizens.[5] And in

Brussels, scientists reported that daily intake of the trace mineral can ameliorate immune system activities by approximately 80 percent.[6] Selenium deficiencies have been linked to exhaustion, liver problems, arthritis, brittle nails, hair loss, garlic-smelling breath, gastrointestinal disorders, and other problems.

Food sources: meats, grains, chicken, dairy products, Brazil nuts, broccoli, brown rice, seafood, salmon, molasses, onions, garlic, kelp, liver

Zinc

Essential to collagen formation and protein synthesis, zinc is involved in over one hundred biochemical processes, from the stimulation of taste, smell, wound healing, and immunity to the maintenance of thick hair and enhancement of healthy blood sugar levels. Zinc is also regarded as the beautifying mineral, since it plays a vital role in strengthening hair and nails, producing unblemished skin, and maintaining regular menses. Perimenopausal women gain great benefits from zinc, which helps bone-building vitamin D absorption. The most important thing to know about zinc is its critical ratio to copper. The ideal ratio of zinc to copper is eight parts zinc to one part copper. Elevated copper levels and a zinc deficiency have been associated with hyperactivity, attention deficit disorder, violence, and depression. The Pfeiffer Treatment Center in Naperville, Illinois, has found that 80 percent of hyperactive patients and 68 percent of behavior-disordered patients have elevated blood copper levels.[7] Lack of zinc can also produce acne, eczema, sensitive skin, sunburn, headaches, and white spots on the fingernails.

Food sources: egg yolks, meats, poultry, fish, lamb, liver, oysters, sardines, mushrooms, pecans, kelp, pumpkin seeds, sunflower seeds, whole grains

Vanadium

Vanadium helps balance blood sugar levels, and a deficiency is dramatically linked to diabetes. This mineral also builds bones and teeth, promotes cellular metabolism, impedes cholesterol synthesis, and supports reproduction. Vanadium is not easily absorbed. A deficiency is often related to cardiovascular and kidney disease.

Food sources: fish, olives, meat, radishes, snap beans, whole grains

Boron

Vital for calcium, phosphorus, and magnesium metabolism, boron is a bone builder. It also supports brain function and attentiveness because of its role as an estrogenic mineral.

Food sources: apples, carrots, grapes, nuts, pears, leafy green vegetables, grains

Other Important Minerals

A few other less-known minerals are also well worth mentioning. Research points to their importance in oxygenation as well as general overall health, and I typically recommend them to my clients. These minerals are not easily found in the food supply because of soil depletion and so are best taken as a dietary supplement, either in liquid, capsule, or tablet form.

Germanium

Germanium helps body organs attract oxygen and bolsters immune system functions. It ameliorates cellular oxygenation and aids in removing toxins and poisons from the body. Its antiviral and antifungal properties render dangerous pathogens and pollutants harmless.

Gold

Gold boosts immune system functions and vitality. Native Americans recognized its worth in promoting a sense of well-being and longevity, using it to cope with mental ailments. It has been credited with helping many health problems, such as arthritis, despair, obesity, gland function, depression, fear, digestive and circulatory disorders, and other problems. When taken with an aspirin, gold has been shown to be helpful in fighting the pain caused by joint inflammation.

Platinum

Platinum fights disease-causing bacteria, fungus, and viruses. It also can help boost the immune system and alleviates back pain, headaches, nerve and muscle tension, sleeplessness, and lethargy.

Silver

Silver is a powerful antibiotic and immune system booster. It has been linked to fighting 650 disease organisms as well as acne, *Candida*, hemorrhoids, ear infections, rheumatism, athlete's foot, cold and flu, bladder irritation, boils, burns, enlarged prostate, meningitis, eczema, warts, parasites, colitis, pneumonia, shingles, diarrhea, tonsillitis, ringworm, and other problems. A silver deficiency makes the body more susceptible to illness.

Palladium

Palladium is an amazing catalyst that researchers such as Dr. Merrill Garnett are finding can heal cancerous cells. In fact, at the Garnett-McKeen Laboratory in Stony Brook, New York, Dr. Garnett has patented a nontoxic chemotherapeutic agent that features a palladium complex of minerals, vitamins, amino acids, and the antioxidant lipoic acid.[8]

CHAPTER 8

PERSONALIZING 40/30/30: YOUR ANCESTRY, METABOLIC TYPE, AND BLOOD TYPE

AS I'VE SAID BEFORE, NO SINGLE DIET FITS ALL. BUT WITH over half of the American public overweight, obviously the dietary standard of the past two decades—the low-fat, high–complex carbohydrate regime—hasn't worked. The 40/30/30 program is a good place to start because it represents a more balanced approach to eating. To personalize this approach one step further, you may want to take into consideration the factors of ancestry, metabolism, and blood type, which address the variables of biochemical individuality.

ANCESTRY

In the past two hundred years, our cultural evolution has far outpaced our physical evolution. For example, we now venture into environments in outer space and beneath the sea to which we will probably never adapt, regardless of time. But we Americans are travelers, too, on a more earthbound scale. Many of us have descended from northern

European, Mediterranean, African, Asian, or Native American peoples, each having its own extremely distinctive diet. We can reasonably suppose that, to some extent, these various peoples have physically adjusted to their different characteristic foods in various ways and are at their healthiest when eating them. If you belong exclusively to some geographic or ethnic group with a characteristic diet, it will probably be beneficial to you to adjust the 40/30/30 plan to fit that diet.

Many of us whose families have been in the United States for more than a generation have mixed ancestry and do not belong exclusively to any particular group. If you are such a person, do not pay too much attention to the ancestry issue, unless you feel distinctly physically better when you eat mostly one kind of food. If that food turns out to belong to some group with which you have no ancestral connection, don't worry. Enjoy it.

METABOLIC TYPE

Many people who tend to put on weight easily belong to one of two metabolic types—they are either slow burners or fast burners. Because of underactive adrenal and thyroid glands, slow burners don't digest and absorb food quickly enough. They tend to favor simple sugars, sweet foods, processed carbohydrates, and soda. They binge on starchy foods. Often having a poor appetite, they dislike protein-rich and fat-rich foods. Slow burners frequently have poor circulation, low blood pressure, and dry skin.

Slow burners need to pay particular attention to proteins and, to a lesser extent, carbohydrates in their diet. Increased dietary protein can increase their metabolic rate by almost one-third. Slow burners should consume animal protein from lean sources (such as tuna, cod, poultry, and eggs) at two meals each day.

Fast burners have overactive adrenal and thyroid glands, and they tend to convert food to blood sugar too speedily. Lacking enough fat and protein in their diet, they often feel hyper, anxious, or irritable, with emotional peaks and valleys corresponding to energy highs and lows. Fast burners frequently feel warm, have high-normal to high blood pressure, and perspire readily.

Fast burners need more fats and protein in their food. They need to eat heavier meats, such as venison, beef, and lamb, or cold-water fish at every meal. The fats in these foods help slow down the metabolism of fast burners.

Not everyone belongs in one or the other of these categories. But if you tend to put on weight easily, the chances are good that you do.

You can discover your metabolic type through hair analysis. However, answering the following quizzes should give you a good idea of your metabolic type. Answer either yes or no to each question.

Slow Burner Quiz

1. Do people regard you as restrained and even tempered?
   Yes ❑   No ❑
2. When you eat red meat, does it feel "heavy" in your system?
   Yes ❑   No ❑
3. Do you prefer to tackle problems one at a time?
   Yes ❑   No ❑
4. Can you skip breakfast without getting hungry or feeling a loss of energy? Yes ❑   No ❑
5. Do you feel a quick pickup from candy, fruit, and other sweet things? Yes ❑   No ❑
6. Do you prefer a "light" meal (for example, salad or pasta) to a "heavy" meal (for example, red meat)? Yes ❑   No ❑
7. Do you become thirsty frequently? Yes ❑   No ❑
8. Do foods such as butter, cheese, and avocados make you feel sluggish? Yes ❑   No ❑
9. Do you need coffee each morning? Yes ❑   No ❑
10. Do you like spicy foods and use condiments such as mustard, ketchup, and salsa? Yes ❑   No ❑

Fast Burner Quiz

1. Do people regard you as high strung or hyperactive?
   Yes ❑ No ❑

2. Do you feel better after eating red meat than after eating poultry? Yes ❑ No ❑

3. Do you like a "hearty" breakfast (for example, bacon and eggs)? Yes ❑ No ❑

4. Under stress, do you reach for salty snacks such as nuts or potato chips? Yes ❑ No ❑

5. Do full-fat dairy products, cheese sauces, and avocados give you a feeling of satisfaction? Yes ❑ No ❑

6. Does eating a full meal every three or fours hours make you feel better? Yes ❑ No ❑

7. When you eat sweet foods, do you feel an energy boost and then an energy loss? Yes ❑ No ❑

8. Do you have an excellent appetite? Yes ❑ No ❑

9. After drinking coffee, do you feel nervous or anxious?
   Yes ❑ No ❑

10. Does butter on toast give you more satisfaction than preserves? Yes ❑ No ❑

Results

If you answered yes to eight or more questions in either quiz, you are a classic slow or fast burner, whichever applies.

As stated earlier, fast burners gain the greatest benefits from the 40/30/30 diet. Slow burners need to adjust the fats downward and the carbs upward.

If you don't have a weight problem and scored somewhere between slow and fast burners—and are therefore neither—you may already be on the diet most suitable for your body type. You may even be, unknowingly, on your own version of the 40/30/30 diet!

BLOOD TYPE

Looking back at how human beings evolved has raised some interesting issues for nutritional researchers. One of the most interesting and important of these issues is how the four major human blood types evolved and how each represents a somewhat different kind of metabolism. Among the leading researchers into this is the naturopathic physician Dr. Peter J. D'Adamo, who has published a recent book on the subject.[1]

The general thinking is that as humans underwent major changes in their efforts to survive in challenging environments, certain chance genetic changes proved advantageous in new environments. Individuals with that genetic change survived better than other people in the new environment. Let's look at how this applies to blood types.

- *Type O.* Regarded as the oldest blood type, at its peak when humans were at the nomadic hunter–gatherer stage, about 40,000 B.C.
- *Type A.* Thought to have emerged when humans became settled in agricultural communities, from about 25,000 to 15,000 B.C. Clearly a change of diet is involved in changing from nomadic hunter–gatherer to settled farmer, and having blood of type A was advantageous for people making that change. If it had not been advantageous, individuals with the new blood type, A, would not have thrived and left descendants.
- *Type B.* Emerged between 15,000 and 10,000 B.C. in the Himalayas. With the later expansion of nomadic people over the Eurasian plains, this blood type became more widespread. It's important to understand that type A didn't gradually merge with or fade into type B. Type B was a sudden genetic change that provided those who possessed it with an advantage in a new lifestyle. That's how evolution works through natural selection. We have to assume there were changes that did not prove

advantageous; descendants of people with those changes no longer exist.

- *Type AB.* The newest blood group. It seems to have evolved about ten to twelve centuries ago, in times of new migrations, conquest, and trade.

But what does all this have to do with Americans today? Am I suggesting, for instance, that something of hunter–gatherers still lingers in people with type O, the commonest blood type today? Yes, I am. Type O people have some remnants or characteristics of the ancient hunter–gatherer type of metabolism. I see evidence that our early progenitors passed on metabolic characteristics to us along with their four bloodlines. If they could pass on differences in blood through genes, they could certainly also pass on differences in digestion and absorption of nutrients. No one argues about that. The question is whether the four blood types also represent typical metabolic differences. The evidence is very strong that this is so.

Type O

A high-protein, low-carbohydrate diet suited type O people for the intense physical activity of hunting. They ate a lot of meat, fish, and whatever wild plants they could. Ideally, lean proteins (free of artificial hormones, antibiotics, and preservatives) should be their prime source. Modern-day individuals with this blood type tend to feel that their bodies do not process foods that developed in the later agricultural stage. These foods typically include dairy products, grains, and legumes. These are the foods type Os should cut back on for optimum health and in order to lose weight.

People with type O blood are generally well suited to the 40/30/30 plan and need to make appropriate substitutions for dairy products, whole wheat, and beans.

Type A

While a typical type O is a meat eater, a typical type A thrives on a vegetarian or near vegetarian diet. Type A people need to ensure that their diet is balanced and that they are ingesting enough protein, vitamins, and minerals. About the only thing people with type A blood have in common with type O people is poor digestion of dairy products. Cutting back on red meat and dairy products helps type A people lose weight. A more vegetarian version of the 40/30/30 program is in order for people with type A blood.

Type B

People with type B blood digest almost all kinds of foods, including fermented dairy products such as yogurt and cottage cheese, very well. For weight loss, D'Adamo recommends that people with type B blood cut back particularly on food containing corn, lentils, peanuts, sesame seeds, and wheat. The 40/30/30 diet is ideally suited for individuals with type B blood.

Type AB

People with the uncommon blood type AB resemble type A people in many respects, except that they can often digest dairy products such as yogurt and cottage cheese without any difficulty. To lose weight, people with type AB blood should cut back on red meat. People with this blood type can use a semivegetarian modification of the 40/30/30 program.

CHAPTER 9

THE 40/30/30 GENERAL GUIDELINES

ON THIS DIET, YOU ARE PERMITTED—IN FACT, REQUIRED—to eat three meals a day *plus* two snacks. The snacks, as well as the meals, should be composed of 40 percent carbohydrate, 30 percent fat, and 30 percent protein. Women often find it beneficial to consume a total of about 1,500 calories daily. Of course, you may need even fewer calories if you are a sedentary, petite woman, in which case I suggest that you look at the 1,200-calorie plan. However, if you are a very active, large man, you should look at the 1,800-calorie plan. But remember, most health experts agree that dropping below 1,200 calories each day could compromise your health.

You can expect to lose about one to two pounds per week, which represents a safe weight-loss rate. Some individuals also lose water weight (from four to seven pounds) during the first week on the diet because of the reduction in carbohydrates. High-carbohydrate diets are notorious for creating fluid retention, especially among women.

GETTING DOWN TO THE BASICS

The 40/30/30 diet plan is simple and gratifying. With this diet you won't feel like you're conducting a complicated chemistry experiment. Instead, you'll have enjoyable meals and snacks without having to bother with scientifically precise measurements. And that's important, because when you become overanxious or compulsive about details, stress sets in and ultimately affects your health.

Much like cooking, putting together a successful diet regimen takes some skill and experience. So at the beginning, keep things simple by following the basic outlines. Then go ahead and let your individual sense of style, food preferences, and personality shape your diet as much as possible—keeping within the suggested boundaries, of course. The more your meals are designed to your specific liking, the more pleasurable they will be *and* the greater the chance you will have of reaching your weight-loss goals.

Now here are some basic pointers, snack foods, and dining out tips to get you started on a rewarding diet lifestyle journey.

THE 40/30/30 FUNDAMENTALS

For each serving of protein (lean meat, poultry, or fish), eat at least one cup of vegetables plus a large salad and, if you wish, half a fruit, along with an unsaturated fat, such as olive oil or nuts.

- Eat up to six ounces of protein at any one meal—roughly equal to the size of the palm of your hand.
- Eat a variety of low-glycemic, fiber-rich vegetables and fruits.
- Avoid simple sugars. Cut down on processed carbohydrates (such as white rice and bagels) high-glycemic, starchy vegetables (such as potatoes and corn), and bread.
- Eat at least a teaspoon of fat at each meal and at snack time (unless you're snacking on nuts) for satiety and blood sugar balance. Try olive oil on your salads and almonds as a snack.
- Drink at least eight to ten 8-ounce glasses of water a day. Be sure to drink more when you are exercising.

- Skip the caffeine. Avoid coffee, tea, and soda.
- Limit alcohol consumption. Have only one drink per day (such as four ounces of wine) and consider it as one carbohydrate serving.
- Eat regularly. Never skip a meal, including snacks. Eat at least every four or five hours while awake. And have a snack before going to bed.
- Eat within one hour of waking.
- Exercise regularly.
- Go easy. Since the 40/30/30 phenomenon will become part of a long-term lifestyle change, don't be in a hurry. Ease into it by making small changes until they become an integral part of your daily life. Remember, it's the change in balanced body chemistry that keeps you on your weight-loss track—not willpower.

40/30/30 FRIENDLY SNACKS

You'll find plenty of tasty snacks in the sample menus in the next chapter. But here are just a few healthy alternatives to keep in mind when you're on the go.

1	cup plain low-fat yogurt
⅓	cup low-fat cottage cheese with either 1 apple, 1 orange, 1 pineapple ring, or 2 rye krisp crackers
1	high-protein muffin (made with soy protein or whey)
1	tablespoon peanut butter on celery
5 to 7	almonds

40/30/30 EATING OUT TIPS

Dining out has always been a challenge to anyone following a diet plan. You have to make rapid decisions while looking at the menu—and then make visual estimates when the food arrives at the table. Here are some pointers on how to stay in control of what you eat.

- According to Marian Burros, servings at American restaurants are much too large and growing even more generous.[1] Before starting to eat, make a visual estimate of what you need and stick to it. Take home the rest if it tastes really good.

- Remember to eyeball your portion of lean meat, poultry, or fish—it should be about the size of your palm.
- Avoid cream sauces and gravies.
- Your portion of cooked vegetables should be about the size of a full coffee mug.
- A small dinner roll is about the size of a plum.
- Make your salad large.
- Order salad dressing on the side and use it sparingly.
- If you have starchy vegetables (such as potatoes) or processed carbohydrates (such as rice or pasta) on your plate, eat very little of them or none at all.
- Eat fresh fruit for dessert.

One last thing to keep in mind: Unless you know people well, it's usually best to keep what you are doing to yourself. People who should be dieting but aren't may feel offended by others who laud their diet regimen. Sit back and be content with the compliments on how good you look.

CHAPTER 10

CREATING YOUR
40/30/30 PHENOMENON

ARE YOU READY TO BEGIN YOUR 40/30/30 JOURNEY TOWARD vibrant well-being and successful weight loss? With this simplified version of the Zone approach, you can enjoy nutritiously balanced meals and snacks without having to figure out the food blocks, made popular in Dr. Barry Sears's benchmark work, *The Zone*. For many, food blocks can be confusing, hard to determine, and too complicated to factor into your regular routine. For simplicity, I therefore use the easier-to-understand, more conventional exchange lists for food choices, portions, and their equivalents in menu planning.

To make things even more simple, this chapter has very basic, easy-to-fix sample menus for your specific daily caloric needs: 1,200, 1,500, or 1,800 calories. Most women who need to lose weight should follow the 1,200-calorie plan, while men can start at 1,500 calories. Women can then graduate to either 1,500 or 1,800 calories, while men can progress to 1,800 calories pretty quickly. And if some of the menu suggestions don't appeal to you, all you have to do is check out the 40/30/30 Friendly Exchanges at the end of this chapter to find tasty substitutes in that particular food group.

Another alternative is to take your 40/30/30 experience to the twenty-first-century tech arena and use Zone Balance software (see Resources). Not only is this program user friendly, but it is certainly the most accurate way to maintain the originally designed 40/30/30 balance of carbohydrate, protein, and fat. Zone Balance does the work for you by calculating grams, blocks, and calories. The program gives you a lot of help, such as letting you know if meals or snacks are in balance and how to bring them in balance if they're not. What I especially like about the software is that you can plug in everyday food selections—and you don't need a Ph.D. in math to use it.

FAT-ZAPPING SUPPLEMENTS

No matter how you decide to calculate your ratios, for even better results you may want to consider augmenting your diet journey with nutritional supplements and fat burners. Many of my clients have enjoyed continued good health and fat-burning success by incorporating dietary supplements into their 40/30/30 plan. My clients and readers have been ordering the supplements described in the following chart from Uni Key Health Systems for many years (see Resources).

Supplement	Recommended Dosage
Uni Key Female Formula (copper free)	2 with breakfast, lunch, and dinner
Uni Key Male Formula (iron free)*	1 with breakfast, lunch, and dinner
Uni Key Weight Loss Formula	2 times daily with meals
Uni Key CLA	1,000 mg/3 times daily (before each meal)
Ultra H-3	1 upon arising and 1 midafternoon

* This supplement may also be used by postmenopausal women.

The supplements described in the following chart will also help boost your 40/30/30 experience. You'll find them at your local health food store.

Supplement	Recommended Dosage
Co-Q10	30 mg/3 times daily with meals
L-carnitine	1,000 mg/2–3 times daily between meals
Neuromin's or Health from the Sun Ultra DHA	200 mg/1–2 times daily with meals

If you're concerned about getting the right fats because you don't like eating fish or oils, nuts, and seeds, add the supplements described in the following chart to your dietary regimen.

Supplement	Recommended Dosage
Super MaxEPA	1,000 mg/2–3 times daily with meals
Flaxseed oil	1 tablespoon or 12 capsules daily
GLA 90	2–4 softgels daily
	or borage oil, 500 mg/1 per meal daily
	or evening primrose oil, 500 mg/2–4 per meal daily
	or black currant seed oil, 90 mg/ 4 times daily with meals

SAMPLE MENUS

Perhaps the quickest and easiest way to get into the 40/30/30 phenomenon is by following the weeklong menu samples that follow. They will give you a sense of how the diet system works. Later, you can let your creativity and individuality take over to design a wider array of meal plan ideas. Simply choose the daily calorie intake for your needs and follow the meal plan. And don't forget to check the 40/30/30 Friendly Exchanges at the end of the chapter for some additional substitutes.

1,200-Calorie Menu

Monday

Breakfast
½ tablespoon olive oil
1 whole egg
3 egg whites
½ cup sliced mushrooms
¼ cup diced celery
   dash of cayenne pepper
½ whole wheat English muffin, toasted
½ cup strawberries

Scramble egg and egg whites in oil with mushrooms, celery, and pepper. Serve with muffin and strawberries.

Midmorning snack
¼ cup low-fat cottage cheese
½ cup pineapple chunks
½ teaspoon flaxseed oil

Mix cottage cheese with pineapple and oil to serve.

Lunch

    2   cups romaine lettuce, torn into bite-sized pieces
    3   ounces broiled skinless chicken breast, cubed
    ¼   cup chopped tomatoes
    ¼   cup cucumber slices
    ½   cup black beans, cooked
    ½   tablespoon sesame oil
    1   tablespoon fresh lemon juice
    1   slice Ezekiel 4:9 sprouted bread, toasted
    1   teaspoon almond butter

Top lettuce with chicken, tomatoes, cucumber, and beans. Drizzle with oil and lemon juice. Serve with bread spread with almond butter.

Midafternoon snack

    3   celery stalks
    ½   tablespoon peanut butter
    ½   tablespoon raisins

Fill stalks with peanut butter and raisins to serve.

Dinner

    2   teaspoons olive oil
    5   ounces shrimp, shelled and deveined
    ¼   cup zucchini, sliced
    ¼   cup onions, sliced
    ¼   cup carrots, sliced
    ½   cup snow peas
    ½   cup mung bean noodles, cooked

Sauté shrimp in oil. Steam vegetables. Serve shrimp over steamed vegetables and mung bean noodles. Add herbs and spices to taste if desired.

Tuesday

Breakfast

BREAKFAST SHAKE:

- ½ cup blueberries
- 8 ounces almond milk
- 1 scoop unflavored whey protein powder
- ½ tablespoon flaxseed oil

Place ingredients in blender and blend until rich and creamy.

Midmorning snack

- 1 slice pumpernickel bread, toasted
- 1 tablespoon tahini

Spread tahini over bread.

Lunch

- 3 ounces tuna, canned in water
- 1 tablespoon Spectrum Natural organic mayonnaise
- ¼ cup diced celery
- ¼ cup diced leeks
- ½ teaspoon curry powder
- 1 whole wheat pita bread, split
- ½ kiwi

Mix tuna with mayonnaise, celery, leeks, and curry powder. Place in pita bread. Enjoy with kiwi.

Midafternoon snack

½ nectarine, sliced
1 tablespoon granola
½ cup plain, unsweetened, low-fat yogurt
1 teaspoon flaxseed oil

Mix nectarine with granola, yogurt, and oil.

Dinner

½ cup canned lentil soup
3 ounces lamb chop
1 teaspoon olive oil
   rosemary
½ cup broccoli florets
¼ cup cauliflower florets
¼ cup kale

Heat lentil soup. Broil chop brushed with oil and rosemary. Steam vegetables. Serve with lamb chop and lentil soup.

Wednesday

Breakfast

¾ cup low-fat cottage cheese

2 tablespoons toasted wheat germ

½ tablespoon flaxseed oil

1 grapefruit

Mix cottage cheese with wheat germ and oil. Serve with grapefruit.

Midmorning snack

½ Granny Smith apple

½ ounce Gouda cheese

Lunch

1 cup spinach

½ cup kidney beans

¼ cup mung bean sprouts

¼ cup mushrooms

2 tablespoons pine nuts

1 tablespoon apple cider vinegar

½ tablespoon fresh lemon juice

1 turkey hot dog, broiled

Dijon mustard

Mix the spinach with beans, sprouts, mushrooms, and pine nuts. Drizzle with vinegar and lemon juice. Serve with hot dog and mustard.

Midafternoon snack

½ high-protein muffin

1 teaspoon flaxseed oil

Drizzle muffin with oil.

Dinner

½ cup cooked whole wheat pasta

½ tablespoon olive oil

1 tablespoon fresh lemon juice

5 ounces broiled salmon

½ cup winter squash, cooked with cinnamon

Toss pasta with oil and lemon juice. Serve with salmon and squash.

Thursday

Breakfast

1   tablespoon part skim ricotta cheese
2   tablespoons salsa
½   tablespoon flaxseed oil
½   whole wheat English muffin, toasted
2   poached eggs

Mix cheese, salsa, and oil together for muffin spread. Serve with eggs.

Midmorning snack

1   peach
4   walnut halves

Lunch

2   cups romaine lettuce, torn into bite-sized pieces
⅛   cup chopped black olives
1   ounce sardines
½   cup cooked beets
½   cup chickpeas
½   tablespoon sesame oil
2   tablespoons fresh lemon juice
1   corn tortilla

Mix lettuce with olives, sardines, beets, and chickpeas. Drizzle with oil and lemon juice. Serve with warmed tortilla.

Midafternoon snack

½ cup low-fat cottage cheese
½ cup cubed cantaloupe
2 rice crackers

Top cottage cheese with cantaloupe. Serve with crackers.

Dinner

CUCUMBER SOUP:

1 cup plain, unsweetened, low-fat yogurt
2 cups diced cucumber
1 teaspoon dill weed

2 rye crisp crackers
3 ounces broiled hamburger with garlic

Mix yogurt, cucumber, and dill weed thoroughly and chill. Serve with crackers and hamburger.

Friday

Breakfast
- ¼ cup chopped tomatoes
- ¼ cup crumbled feta cheese
  fresh basil
- 2 teaspoons grated Parmesan cheese
- ½ teaspoon olive oil
- 1 small whole wheat pita bread, split

Mix tomatoes, feta cheese, basil, Parmesan cheese, and olive oil together. Fill pita bread with mixture to serve.

Midmorning snack
- 1 slice Ezekiel 4:9 bread, toasted
- 1 tablespoon peanut butter
- ½ cup honeydew melon, cubed

Spread bread with peanut butter to serve with melon.

Lunch
- ½ tablespoon olive oil
- 3 ounces tofu, cubed
- ¼ cup each red, yellow, green, and orange peppers, diced
- ⅛ cup onion, finely chopped
- ¼ cup water chestnuts, sliced
- ¼ cup bok choy, chopped
- ½ cup rice noodles, cooked

Stir-sauté the tofu in oil. Steam peppers, onion, water chestnuts, and bok choy. Serve tofu and vegetables over rice noodles. Add herbs and sprouts to taste.

Midafternoon snack

10 grapes

½ ounce cheddar cheese

2 rye crisp crackers

Dinner

3 ounces ground turkey

½ teaspoon fennel

1 teaspoon sesame oil

½ cup tomato sauce

½ cup broccoli florets

½ cup cauliflower florets

½ cup brown rice, cooked

Brown turkey and fennel in oil. Add tomato sauce amd simmer. Steam vegetables. Serve turkey mixture over steamed vegetables and rice.

Saturday

Breakfast

½ small whole wheat bagel, toasted

½ ounce mozzarella cheese, part skim, low moisture

1 slice tomato

Top bagel with cheese and tomato to serve.

Midmorning snack

3 dried prunes

3 walnut halves

Lunch

2 cups romaine lettuce, torn into bite-sized pieces

4 ounces broiled chicken breast, cubed

¼ cup diced tomatoes

¼ cup chopped mushrooms

1 tablespoon fresh lemon juice

½ tablespoon flaxseed oil

½ whole wheat pita bread

Mix lettuce with chicken, tomatoes, and mushrooms. Drizzle with lemon juice and oil. Serve with pita bread.

Midafternoon snack

1   ounce smoked salmon
2   rye crisp crackers

Dinner

3   ounces halibut
1   teaspoon fresh lemon juice
½   garlic clove, minced
½   cup cooked parsnips
1   teaspoon flaxseed oil
¾   cup brown rice, cooked

Brush halibut with lemon juice and garlic before broiling. Drizzle parsnips with oil. Serve fish with parsnips and rice.

Sunday

Breakfast

1 Granny Smith apple

1 teaspoon apple juice

1 tablespoon raisins

¼ teaspoon cinnamon

½ teaspoon flaxseed oil

Bake apple with apple juice, raisins, and cinnamon. Drizzle with flaxseed oil before serving.

Midmorning snack

1 slice rye bread, toasted

1 tablespoon tahini

Spread tahini over bread.

Lunch

2 cups spinach leaves

2 hard-cooked eggs, sliced

2 ounces smoked salmon

⅛ cup diced celery

½ cup artichoke hearts, chopped

¼ cup red pepper, diced

1 tablespoon apple cider vinegar

1 teaspoon olive oil

Mix spinach leaves with eggs, salmon, celery, artichoke hearts, and pepper. Drizzle with vinegar and olive oil to serve.

Midafternoon snack

½ ounce almonds

1 medium plum

Dinner

4 ounces cod

1 teaspoon olive oil

   parsley

½ cup broccoli florets

½ cup asparagus

½ medium baked potato

¼ cup low-fat cottage cheese

1 teaspoon flaxseed oil

Brush cod with parsley and oil before baking. Steam vegetables.
Serve cod with vegetables and baked potato topped with cottage
cheese and flaxseed oil.

1,500-Calorie Menu

Monday

Breakfast

- ½ tablespoon olive oil
- 1 whole egg
- 3 egg whites
- ½ cup sliced mushrooms, steamed
- ¼ cup diced celery, steamed
   dash of cayenne pepper
- ½ tablespoon nut butter
- ½ whole wheat English muffin, toasted
- ½ cup strawberries

Scramble egg and egg whites in olive oil. Add steamed mushrooms and celery and cayenne. Spread nut butter over muffin. Serve with strawberries.

Midmorning snack

- ¼ cup low-fat cottage cheese
- ¼ cup pineapple chunks
- ½ teaspoon flaxseed oil

Mix cottage cheese, pineapple, and flaxseed oil together before serving.

Lunch

- 2 cups romaine lettuce, torn into bite-sized pieces
- 6 ounces broiled, skinless chicken breast, cubed, with tarragon
- 1 tablespoon Parmesan cheese

¼ cup chopped tomatoes
¼ cup cucumber slices
½ tablespoon flaxseed oil
1 tablespoon fresh lemon juice
1 slice Ezekiel 4:9 sprouted bread, toasted
½ tablespoon unsweetened fruit preserves

Mix lettuce with chicken, cheese, tomatoes, and cucumbers. Drizzle oil and lemon juice over salad. Spread bread with preserves and serve.

Midafternoon snack

4 celery stalks
1 tablespoon peanut butter

Dinner

2 teaspoons olive oil
5 ounces shrimp, shelled and deveined
½ cup zucchini, sliced
¼ cup onions, diced
½ cup carrots, chopped
½ cup snow peas
¾ cup mung bean noodles, cooked

Sauté shrimp in oil. Steam vegetables and serve wth shrimp over noodles.

Tuesday

Breakfast

BREAKFAST SHAKE:

- ¾ cup blueberries
- 8 ounces almond milk
- 1 scoop unflavored whey protein powder
- 1 tablespoon flaxseed oil

Place all ingredients in blender and blend until rich and creamy.

Midmorning snack

- 1 slice pumpernickel bread, toasted
- 1 tablespoon tahini
- 1 tablespoon raisins

Spread bread with tahini and top with raisins.

Lunch

- 5 ounces tuna, canned in water
- 1½ tablespoons Spectrum Natural organic mayonnaise
- ¼ cup celery, diced
- ¼ cup leeks, diced
- ½ teaspoon curry powder
- 1 whole wheat pita bread, split
- 1 kiwi

Mix tuna with mayonnaise, celery, leeks, and curry powder. Place in pita bread. Serve with kiwi.

Midafternoon snack

- 1   nectarine, sliced
- 1   tablespoon granola
- ½   cup plain, unsweetened, low-fat yogurt
- 1   teaspoon flaxseed oil

Mix nectarine with granola, yogurt, and flaxseed oil to serve.

Dinner

- 1   cup canned lentil soup
- 4   ounces lamb chop
- 1   teaspoon olive oil
- ½   cup broccoli florets
- ½   cup cauliflower florets
- ½   cup kale

Heat lentil soup. Brush lamb chop with oil before broiling. Steam vegetables. Serve with lamb chop and lentil soup.

Wednesday

Breakfast
¾ cup low-fat cottage cheese

2 tablespoons toasted wheat germ

1 tablespoon flaxseed oil

1 grapefruit

Mix cottage cheese with wheat germ and oil. Serve with grapefruit.

Midmorning snack
1 Granny Smith apple

½ ounce Gouda cheese

2 rye crisp crackers

Lunch
2 cups spinach leaves

½ cup kidney beans, cooked

¼ cup bean sprouts

¼ cup mushrooms

1 tablespoon pine nuts

1 tablespoon apple cider vinegar

1 tablespoon lemon juice

½ teaspoon flaxseed oil

2 turkey hot dogs, broiled

Dijon mustard

Mix spinach leaves with beans, sprouts, mushrooms, and pine nuts. Drizzle with vinegar, lemon juice, and oil. Serve along with hot dogs and mustard.

Midafternoon snack

1   high-protein muffin
1   teaspoon flaxseed oil

Drizzle oil over muffin before serving.

Dinner

½   cup whole wheat pasta, cooked
½   tablespoon olive oil
1   tablespoon fresh lemon juice
5   ounces broiled salmon with dill
½   cup winter squash, cooked with cinnamon

Toss pasta with olive oil and lemon juice. Serve with salmon and squash.

Thursday

Breakfast
- ½ whole wheat English muffin, toasted
- 2 tablespoons part skim ricotta cheese
- 2 tablespoons salsa
- 2 poached eggs

Top muffin with cheese and salsa and serve with eggs.

Midmorning snack
- 1 peach
- 5 walnut halves

Lunch
- 2 cups romaine lettuce, torn into bite-sized pieces
- ¼ cup black olives, chopped
- ¼ cup beets, cooked
- 2 ounces sardines
- ½ cup chickpeas
- ½ tablespoon sesame oil
- 2 tablespoons fresh lemon juice
- 1 corn tortilla

Mix lettuce with olives, beets, sardines, and chickpeas. Drizzle with oil and lemon juice. Serve with warmed tortilla.

Midafternoon snack

¾ cup low-fat cottage cheese

1 cup cantaloupe, cubed

2 rice crackers

Top cottage cheese with cantaloupe and serve with crackers.

Dinner

CUCUMBER SOUP:

1 cup plain, unsweetened, low-fat yogurt

2 cups cucumber, diced

1 teaspoon dill weed

3 ounces broiled hamburger with garlic

½ whole wheat English muffin, toasted

½ teaspoon unsweetened fruit preserves

Mix yogurt, cucumber, and dill weed thoroughly and chill. Serve with hamburger and muffin spread with preserves.

Friday

Breakfast

¼ cup chopped tomatoes
¼ cup crumbled feta cheese
   fresh basil
2 teaspoons grated Parmesan cheese
½ teaspoon olive oil
1 small whole wheat pita bread, split

Mix tomatoes, feta cheese, basil, Parmesan cheese, and olive oil together for filling pita bread.

Midmorning snack

1 slice Ezekiel 4:9 bread, toasted
1 tablespoon peanut butter
1 cup honeydew melon, cubed or balled

Spread bread with peanut butter and serve with melon.

Lunch

½ tablespoon olive oil
4 ounces tofu, cubed
¼ cup each red, yellow, green, and orange peppers, diced
⅛ cup onion, chopped
¼ cup water chestnuts, sliced
¼ cup bok choy, chopped
½ cup rice noodles, cooked

Stir-sauté tofu in oil. Steam peppers, onion, water chestnuts, and bok choy. Combine tofu and vegetables and serve over noodles. Add herbs and spices to taste.

Midafternoon snack

10 grapes

½ ounce cheddar cheese

2 rye crisp crackers

Dinner

1 teaspoon sesame oil

5 ounces ground turkey

1 teaspoon fennel

¾ cup tomato sauce

½ cup broccoli florets

½ cup cauliflower florets

¾ cup brown rice, cooked

Brown turkey and fennel in oil. Add tomato sauce and simmer. Steam broccoli and cauliflower. Serve turkey mixture over steamed vegetables and rice.

Saturday

Breakfast
½ small whole wheat bagel, toasted
½ ounce part skim, low-moisture mozzarella cheese
1 slice tomato

Top bagel with cheese and tomato.

Midmorning snack
3 dried prunes
3 walnut halves

Lunch
2 cups romaine lettuce, torn into bite-sized pieces
6 ounces broiled skinless chicken breast, cubed
¼ cup diced tomatoes
¼ cup chopped mushrooms
1 tablespoon fresh lemon juice
½ tablespoon flaxseed oil
½ whole wheat pita bread

Mix lettuce with chicken, tomatoes, and mushrooms. Drizzle with lemon juice and oil. Serve with pita bread.

Midafternoon snack

1½ ounces smoked salmon
4 whole grain rye crackers

Dinner

5 ounces halibut
1 teaspoon fresh lemon juice
1 garlic clove, minced
½ cup parsnips, cooked
1 teaspoon flaxseed oil
¾ cup brown rice, cooked

Brush halibut with lemon juice and minced garlic before broiling. Drizzle parsnips with oil. Serve fish with parsnips and rice.

Sunday

Breakfast
 1 Granny Smith apple
 1 teaspoon apple juice
 2 tablespoons raisins
 ¼ teaspoon cinnamon
 ½ teaspoon flaxseed oil

Bake apple with juice, raisins, and cinnamon. Drizzle with oil before serving.

Midmorning snack
 1 slice rye bread, toasted
 1 tablespoon tahini

Spread bread with tahini before serving.

Lunch
 2 cups spinach leaves
 2 hard-cooked eggs, sliced
 4 ounces smoked salmon
 ⅛ cup celery, diced
 ½ cup artichoke hearts, chopped
 ¼ cup red pepper, diced
 ½ tablespoon apple cider vinegar
 ½ tablespoon fresh lemon juice
 1 tablespoon olive oil

Mix spinach with eggs, salmon, celery, artichoke, and pepper. Drizzle with vinegar, lemon juice, and oil to serve.

Midafternoon snack

½ ounce almonds

1 medium plum

Dinner

5 ounces cod

1 tablespoon olive oil

parsley

½ cup broccoli florets

½ cup asparagus

1 medium baked potato

½ cup low-fat cottage cheese

Brush cod with oil and parsley before baking. Steam vegetables. Serve fish with vegetables and potato topped with cottage cheese.

1,800-Calorie Menu

Monday

Breakfast

½ teaspoon olive oil
2 whole eggs
4 egg whites
1 whole wheat English muffin, toasted
1 tablespoon nut butter
1 cup strawberries

Scramble eggs and egg whites in oil. Spread muffin with nut butter and serve with strawberries.

Midmorning snack

½ cup low-fat cottage cheese
½ cup pineapple chunks
1 teaspoon flaxseed oil

Mix cottage cheese with pineapple and flaxseed oil to serve.

Lunch

2 cups romaine lettuce, torn into bite-sized pieces
6 ounces broiled skinless chicken breast, cubed
1 tablespoon Parmesan cheese
¼ cup tomatoes, chopped
¼ cup cucumber slices
½ tablespoon flaxseed oil
2 tablespoons fresh lemon juice

2   slices Ezekiel 4:9 sprouted bread, toasted
1   tablespoon unsweetened fruit preserves

Mix lettuce with chicken, cheese, tomatoes, and cucumber. Drizzle with oil and lemon juice. Spread bread with preserves and serve with salad.

Midafternoon snack

4   celery stalks
1   tablespoon peanut butter
1   tablespoon raisins

Fill stalks with peanut butter and raisins to serve.

Dinner

2   teaspoons olive oil
5   ounces shrimp, shelled and deveined
½   cup zucchini, sliced
¼   cup onions, chopped
½   cup carrots, chopped
½   cup snow peas
1   cup mung bean noodles, cooked

Sauté shrimp in oil. Steam vegetables and serve with shrimp over noodles. Add herbs and spices to taste, if desired.

Tuesday

Breakfast

BREAKFAST SHAKE:

¾ cup blueberries

8 ounces almond milk

1 scoop unflavored whey protein powder

1 tablespoon flaxseed oil

1 tablespoon wheat germ, toasted

Place all ingredients except wheat germ in blender and blend until rich and creamy. Top with wheat germ.

Midmorning snack

1 slice pumpernickel bread, toasted

1 tablespoon tahini

2 tablespoons raisins

Spread bread with tahini and top with raisins.

Lunch

6 ounces tuna, canned in water

2 tablespoons Spectrum Natural organic mayonnaise

¼ cup celery, diced

¼ cup leeks, diced

½ teaspoon curry powder

1 whole wheat pita bread, split

1 kiwi

Mix tuna, mayonnaise, celery, leeks, and curry powder together and fill pita bread. Serve with kiwi.

Midafternoon snack

1   nectarine, sliced
2   tablespoons granola
¾   cup plain, unsweetened, low-fat yogurt
½   tablespoon flaxseed oil

Mix nectarine with granola, yogurt, and flaxseed oil to serve.

Dinner

1½ cups canned lentil soup
4   ounces lamb chop
1   teaspoon olive oil
   rosemary
½   cup broccoli florets
½   cup cauliflower florets
½   cup kale

Heat soup. Brush lamb chop with oil and rosemary before broiling. Steam vegetables. Serve with lamb chop and soup.

Wednesday

Breakfast
- 1 cup low-fat cottage cheese
- 2 tablespoons toasted wheat germ
- 1 tablespoon flaxseed oil
- 1 grapefruit

Mix cottage cheese with wheat germ and oil. Serve with grapefruit.

Midmorning snack
- 1 Granny Smith apple
- 1 ounce Gouda cheese
- 4 rye crisp crackers

Lunch
- 2 cups spinach
- 1 cup kidney beans, cooked
- ¼ cup mung bean sprouts
- ¼ cup mushrooms, cooked
- 1 tablespoon pine nuts
- 1 tablespoon apple cider vinegar
- 1 tablespoon lemon juice
- ½ teaspoon flaxseed oil
- 2 turkey hot dogs, broiled
  Dijon mustard

Mix spinach with beans, sprouts, mushrooms, and pine nuts. Drizzle with vinegar, juice, and oil. Serve with hot dogs and mustard.

Midafternoon snack

1   high-protein muffin
1   teaspoon flaxseed oil

Drizzle muffin with oil to serve.

Dinner

½   cup whole wheat pasta, cooked
½   tablespoon olive oil
1   tablespoon fresh lemon juice
6   ounces broiled salmon with dill
¾   cup winter squash, cooked with cinnamon

Toss pasta with olive oil and lemon juice. Serve with salmon and squash.

Thursday

Breakfast

1 whole wheat English muffin, toasted

3 tablespoons part skim ricotta cheese

3 tablespoons salsa

2 poached eggs

Top muffin with cheese and salsa. Serve with the poached eggs.

Midmorning snack

1 peach

6 walnut halves

Lunch

2 cups romaine lettuce, torn into bite-sized pieces

¼ cup chopped black olives

2 ounces sardines

¾ cup beets, cooked

¾ cup chickpeas

½ tablespoon sesame oil

2 tablespoons fresh lemon juice

1 corn tortilla

Mix lettuce with olives, sardines, beets, and chickpeas. Drizzle with oil and lemon juice and serve with warmed tortilla.

Midafternoon snack

¾ cup low-fat cottage cheese

1 cup cantaloupe, cubed

2 rice crackers

Top cottage cheese with cantaloupe and serve with crackers.

Dinner

CUCUMBER SOUP:

1 cup plain, unsweetened, low-fat yogurt

2 cups cucumber, diced

1 teaspoon dill weed

4 ounces broiled hamburger with garlic

½ whole wheat English muffin, toasted

½ teaspoon unsweetened fruit preserves

¼ teaspoon flaxseed oil

Mix yogurt, cucumber, and dill weed thoroughly and chill. Serve with hamburger and muffin, spread with preserves and drizzled with oil.

Friday

Breakfast

¼ cup chopped tomatoes

¼ cup crumbled feta cheese

    fresh basil

2 teaspoons grated Parmesan cheese

½ teaspoon olive oil

1 small whole wheat pita bread, split

Mix tomatoes, feta cheese, basil, Parmesan cheese, and olive oil together. Fill pita bread with mixture and serve.

Midmorning snack

2 slices Ezekiel 4:9 bread, toasted

1½ tablespoons peanut butter

1½ cups honeydew melon, cubed

Spread bread with peanut butter and serve with melon.

Lunch

½ tablespoon olive oil

6 ounces tofu, cubed

¼ cup each red, yellow, green, and orange peppers, diced

⅛ cup onion, chopped

½ cup bok choy, chopped

½ cup rice noodles, cooked

½ cup peas, cooked

Sauté tofu in oil. Steam peppers, onion, and bok choy. Serve tofu and vegetables over rice noodles with peas.

Midafternoon snack

10 grapes

½ ounce cheddar cheese

2 rye crisp crackers

Dinner

5 ounces ground turkey

1 teaspoon fennel

1 teaspoon sesame oil

¾ cup tomato sauce

½ cup broccoli florets

½ cup cauliflower florets

½ cup yellow squash

¾ cup brown rice, cooked

Brown turkey and fennel in oil. Add tomato sauce and simmer. Steam broccoli, cauliflower, and squash. Serve turkey mixture over steamed vegetables and rice.

Saturday

Breakfast

1   small whole wheat bagel, toasted
¾   ounce part skim, low-moisture mozzarella cheese
2   tomato slices

Top bagel with cheese and tomatoes and serve.

Midmorning snack

3   dried prunes
3   walnut halves

Lunch

2   cups romaine lettuce, torn into bite-sized pieces
6   ounces broiled tarragon chicken breast, cubed
¼   cup tomatoes, diced
¼   cup chopped mushrooms
½   cup green beans, cooked
1   tablespoon fresh lemon juice
1   tablespoon flaxseed oil
1   whole wheat pita bread

Mix lettuce with chicken, tomatoes, mushrooms, and green beans.
Drizzle with lemon juice and oil. Serve with pita bread.

Midafternoon snack

2 ounces smoked salmon
6 whole grain rye crackers

Dinner

5 ounces halibut
1 teaspoon fresh lemon juice
1 teaspoon peanut oil
1 garlic clove, minced
½ cup parsnips, cooked
¾ cup brown rice, cooked
½ cup warm asparagus

Brush halibut with lemon juice, oil, and garlic before broiling. Serve fish with parsnips, rice, and asparagus.

Sunday

Breakfast

1 Granny Smith apple
1 teaspoon apple juice
2 tablespoons raisins
¼ teaspoon cinnamon
½ teaspoon flaxseed oil

Bake apple with juice, raisins, and cinnamon. Drizzle with oil and serve.

Midmorning snack

2 slices rye bread
1½ tablespoons tahini

Spread bread with tahini and serve.

Lunch

2 cups spinach leaves
1 hard-cooked egg, sliced
4 ounces smoked salmon
⅛ cup celery, diced
½ cup artichoke hearts, chopped
¼ cup red pepper, diced
½ tablespoon apple cider vinegar
½ tablespoon fresh lemon juice
1 tablespoon peanut oil

Mix spinach with egg, salmon, celery, artichoke hearts, and pepper. Drizzle with vinegar, lemon juice, and oil before serving.

Midafternoon snack

1   ounce almonds
2   medium plums

Dinner

6   ounces cod
½   tablespoon olive oil
    parsley
½   cup broccoli florets
½   cup asparagus
½   cup Brussels sprouts
1   medium baked potato
½   cup low-fat cottage cheese

Brush cod with oil and parsley before baking. Steam vegetables. Serve cod with vegetables and potato topped with cottage cheese.

40/30/30 FRIENDLY EXCHANGES

Looking for a food substitute? Locate the specific food group in which you want to make the exchange, then choose from among the many 40/30/30 friendly alternatives.

40/30/30 Friendly Vegetables

The following vegetables may be substituted for one another for variety and creative menu planning:

Artichoke, medium, cooked	½ cup
Asparagus, cooked	½ cup
Beets, cooked	½ cup
Broccoli, cooked	½ cup
Brussels sprouts, cooked	½ cup
Cabbage, cooked	½ cup
Cauliflower, cooked	½ cup
Daikon, cooked	½ cup
Eggplant, cooked	½ cup
Green beans, cooked	½ cup
Greens, cooked	½ cup
Leafy greens: arugula, chard, dandelion, escarole, kale, mustard, radicchio, red or green leaf lettuce, romaine lettuce, spinach, watercress	1 cup
Mushrooms, cooked	½ cup
Okra, cooked	½ cup
Raw veggies: broccoli, cauliflower, celery, cucumbers, radishes, sprouts, tomatoes	1 cup

Red or green peppers, cooked	½ cup
Snow peas, cooked	½ cup
Summer squash, cooked	½ cup
Zucchini, cooked	½ cup

40/30/30 Starchy Vegetables

The following starchy vegetables, breads, cereals, grains, crackers, flours, legumes, and pastas can be interchanged for one another:

Chestnuts, roasted	4 large or 6 small
Corn, cooked	½ cup
Corn on the cob	1 (4 inches long)
Parsnips, cooked	1 small
Peas, cooked	¼ cup
Potatoes, white (baked or boiled)	1 small
Potatoes, white, mashed	½ cup
Pumpkin, cooked	¾ cup
Rutabaga, cooked	1 small
Squash (winter types), cooked	½ cup
Succotash, cooked	½ cup

40/30/30 Breads

Bagel, whole wheat	½ small
Bread (rye, whole wheat)	1 slice
Breadsticks	4 (7 inches long)
Bun (hamburger or hot dog)	½
Croutons	½ cup
Pancakes (whole grain)	2 (3-inch diameter)
Pita bread	½ of a 6-inch pocket
Tortilla, corn	1 (6-inch tortilla)

40/30/30 Cereals and Grains

Amaranth, cooked	½ cup
Barley, cooked	⅓ cup
Bran flakes	½ cup
Bran (unprocessed rice or wheat)	¼ cup
Buckwheat groats (kasha, cooked)	½ cup
Cornmeal, cooked	⅓ cup
Couscous, cooked	⅓ cup
Grits, cooked	½ cup
Kamut, cooked	½ cup
Millet, cooked	⅔ cup
Oatmeal (steel-cut), cooked	½ cup
Oats, rolled, cooked	½ cup
Quinoa, cooked	⅓ cup
Rice (brown), cooked	⅓ cup
Rice (wild), cooked	⅓ cup
Shredded wheat biscuit	1 large
Spelt, cooked	½ cup
Teff, cooked	⅓ cup
Wheat (bulgur, cracked, rolled)	½ cup
Wheatena, cooked	½ cup
Wheat germ	3 tablespoons

40/30/30 Crackers

Matzoh (whole wheat)	½ matzoh (6 inch or 4 inch)
Pretzels (whole grain)	1 large
Rice wafers (brown rice, Westbrae)	4

Ryvita Light or Dark Crisp Bread	1 to 1½ crackers
Ryvita Original Snack Bread	2 crackers
Ryvita Sesame Snack Bread	2 crackers
Wasa Hearty Crisp Bread	1 cracker
Wasa Light Rye Crisp Bread	2 crackers
Wasa Savory Crisp Bread	2 crackers
Wasa Whole Grain Crisp Bread	2 crackers
Whole wheat crackers (AK-Mak)	4 crackers
Whole wheat crackers (Health Valley)	13 crackers

40/30/30 Flours

Arrowroot	2 tablespoons
Buckwheat	3 tablespoons
Cornmeal	2 tablespoons
Cornstarch	2 tablespoons
Potato flour	2½ tablespoons
Rice flour	3 tablespoons
Soya powder	3 tablespoons
Spelt	3 tablespoons
Whole wheat	3 tablespoons

40/30/30 Legumes

Beans (baked), plain	½ cup
Beans (dried), cooked	½ cup
Lentils (dried), cooked	¼ cup
Peas (dried), cooked	½ cup
Peas (split), cooked	¼ cup

40/30/30 Pastas

Noodles: cooked macaroni or spaghetti	¼ cup
Noodles: rice (cooked)	½ cup
Noodles: whole wheat (cooked)	½ cup
Pasta: whole wheat (cooked)	½ cup

40/30/30 Friendly Fruits

You can use these fruits interchangeably, although the lower glycemic fruits are preferred. (See the glycemic index on pages 12–14.)

Apple	1
Apple butter (sugar free)	2 tablespoons
Apple juice or cider	⅓ cup
Applesauce (unsweetened)	½ cup
Apricots (dried, unsulfured)	4 halves
Apricots (fresh)	3
Banana	½
Berries	½ cup
Cantaloupe	1 cup, cubed
Cherries	12
Dates	2
Figs (dried)	1 small
Figs (fresh)	1 large
Fruit cocktail (canned in juice)	½ cup
Fruit preserves (sugar-free)	2 tablespoons
Grapefruit	½ small
Grapefruit juice	½ cup
Grape juice	¼ cup
Grapes	10
Honeydew melon, cubed	1 cup
Kiwi	1 medium

Lemon	1
Lime	1
Mango, sliced	⅓ cup
Nectarine	1
Orange	1 small
Orange juice (any style)	½ cup
Papaya	½ cup
Peach	1 medium
Peaches, canned	½ cup
Pear	1
Persimmon	1 medium
Pineapple	½ cup
Pineapple juice	⅓ cup
Plums	2
Prune juice	¼ cup
Prunes	2 medium
Raisins	2 tablespoons
Raspberries	⅔ cup
Strawberries	¾ cup
Tangerine	1 large
Watermelon	½ cup

40/30/30 Friendly Fats

Including healthy fats from a variety of sources is especially critical to your weight-loss goals. When using omega-3-rich flaxseed oil, keep in mind that it is sensitive to air, heat, and light and should only be used in no-heat recipes.

Almond butter	1 tablespoon
Almonds, raw, whole	7
Avocado	⅛ medium
Brazil nuts, raw, whole	2

Butter	1 tablespoon
Cashews	5
Cream, half and half	1 tablespoon
Cream, sour	1 tablespoon
Cream cheese	1 tablespoon
Flaxseed oil	1 tablespoon
Grapeseed oil	1 tablespoon
Hazelnuts, raw, whole	3
Macadamia nuts, raw, whole	3
Macadamia oil	1 tablespoon
Mayonnaise (Spectrum Natural organic)	1 tablespoon
Nayonaise (soy based)	1 tablespoon
Olive oil	1 tablespoon
Olives	8
Peanut butter	1 tablespoon
Peanuts	10
Pecans, raw, halves	4
Pine nuts, raw	1 tablespoon
Pistachios	15
Pumpkin seeds, raw	1 tablespoon
Sunflower seeds, raw	1 tablespoon
Tahini	1 tablespoon
Walnuts, raw, halves	4

40/30/30 Friendly Proteins

Lean proteins cover quite a tantalizing array of meats, fish, dairy, and vegetarian alternatives. There's never a reason to get bored or wonder what to eat. Some examples and their equivalents include the following:

Protein: Meat, Poultry, and Eggs

Beef, ground (10 percent or less fat)	3 ounces
Beef, lean cuts (sirloin, top round)	3 ounces
Buffalo	3 ounces
Chicken breast, skinless	3 ounces
Duck	3 ounces
Egg, whites	4
Egg, whole	2
Lamb, lean	3 ounces
Ostrich	3 ounces
Rabbit	3 ounces
Turkey breast, skinless	3 ounces
Turkey, dark meat, skinless	3 ounces
Veal	3 ounces
Venison	3 ounces

Protein: Fish and Seafood

Bass	3 ounces
Bluefish	3 ounces
Calamari	3 ounces
Catfish	3 ounces
Clams	3 ounces
Cod	3 ounces
Crab meat	3 ounces
Haddock	3 ounces
Halibut	3 ounces
Lobster	3 ounces
Mackerel	3 ounces
Orange roughy	3 ounces
Pike, Northern	3 ounces

Salmon	3 ounces
Sardines	3 ounces
Scallops	3 ounces
Shrimp	3 ounces
Snapper	3 ounces
Sole	3 ounces
Swordfish	3 ounces
Trout	3 ounces
Trout, canned in water	3 ounces
Tuna, canned in water	3 ounces
Tuna, steak	3 ounces

Protein: Dairy

Cheese, reduced fat	1 ounce
Cottage cheese, dry curd	½ cup
Cottage cheese, low fat	½ cup
Farmers' cheese	¼ cup
Feta cheese	1 ounce
Gouda cheese	1 ounce
Mozzarella, skim	1 ounce
Parmesan	2 tablespoons
Ricotta, skim	2 ounces or ¼ cup

Protein: Vegetarian

Naturade's Fat Free Vegetable Protein	1 scoop
Solgar's Whey to Go (lactose free)	1 scoop
Tempeh	4 ounces
Tofu	4 ounces

NOTES

INTRODUCTION

1. Jeffrey P. Koplan, "Diabetes: A Serious Public Health Problem," *Centers for Disease Control and Prevention* (2000). www.cdc.gov/diabetes/pubs/glance.htm.
2. Ann Louise Gittleman, *Beyond Pritikin* (New York: Bantam, 1996).
3. M. J. Hamadeh et al., "Nutritional Aspects of Flaxseed in the Human Diet," *Proceedings of the Flax Institute* 4 (1992): 48–53.
4. L. J. Stevens et al., "Essential Fatty Acid Metabolism in Boys with Attention-Deficit Hyperactivity Disorder," *American Journal of Clinical Nutrition* 62, no. 4 (1995): 761–68.

CHAPTER 2

1. Ann Louise Gittleman, *Super Nutrition for Men* (New York: Avery, 1999).

CHAPTER 3

1. Jennie Brand-Miller et al., *The Glucose Revolution: The Authoritative Guide to the Glycemic Index* (New York: Marlowe, 1999).

2. S. Boyd Eaton and Melvin Konner, M.D., "Paleolithic Nutrition: A Consideration of Its Nature and Current Implications," *New England Journal of Medicine* 312, no. 5 (1985): 283–89.
3. Gerald M. Reaven, M.D., *Syndrome X: Overcoming the Silent Killer That Can Give You a Heart Attack* (New York: Simon & Schuster, 2000).
4. Gary Evans, M.D., *Chromium Picolinate* (New York: Avery, 1996), 64.
5. Reaven, *Syndrome X.*
6. Priya Mohanty et al., "Glucose Challenge Stimulates Reactive Oxygen Species (ROS) Generation by Leucocytes," *Journal of Clinical Endocrinology and Metabolism* 85, no. 8 (2000): 2970–73.
7. A. Cerami and M. Brownlee, "Glucose and Aging," *Scientific American* 256 (1987): 90–96; and P. Ulrich and A. Cerami, "Protein Glycation, Diabetes and Aging," *Recent Progressive Hormone Research* 56 (2001): 1–21.
8. Robert Atkins, M.D., *Age-Defying Diet Revolution* (New York: St. Martin's Press, 2000).
9. Gerald M. Reaven, M.D., "Pathophysiology of Insulin Resistance in Human Disease," *Physiological Reviews* 75, no. 3 (1995): 473–85.
10. Jerry Adler and Claudia Kalb, "An American Epidemic: Diabetes," *Newsweek*, 4 September 2000, 40–47.
11. A. H. Mokdad et al., "Diabetes Trends in the U.S.," *Diabetes Care* 23, no. 9 (2000): 1278–83.
12. George Ryan, *Reclaiming Male Sexuality: A Guide to Potency, Vitality, and Prowess* (New York: Evans, 1997).
13. Adler and Kalb, "An American Epidemic."
14. Jeffrey P. Koplan, "Diabetes: A Serious Public Health Problem," *Centers for Disease Control and Prevention* (2000). www.cdc.gov/diabetes/pubs/glance.htm
15. G. A. Colditz et al., "Weight as a Risk Factor for Clinical Diabetes in Women," *American Journal of Epidemiology* 132 (1990): 501–13.
16. J. E. Monson et al., "Physical Activity and Incidence of Non-Insulin-Dependent Diabetes Mellitus in Women," *Lancet* 338, no. 8770 (1991): 774–78.
17. Jorge Salmeron et al., "Dietary Fiber, Glycemic Load, and Risk of Non-Insulin-Dependent Diabetes Mellitus in Women," *Journal of the American Medical Association* 277, no. 6 (February 12, 1967): 472-77.
18. Richard Heller and Rachel Heller, *The Carbohydrate Addicts Diet* (New York: NAL Dutton, 1992).
19. John Yudkin, M.D., *Sweet and Dangerous* (New York: Wyden, 1972).
20. T. L. Cleave, *The Saccharine Disease: The Master Disease of Our Time* (Lincolnwood, Ill.: Keats, 1975).
21. Gerald M. Reaven, M.D., "Resistance to Insulin-Mediated Glucose Disposal as a Predictor of Cardiovascular Disease," *Journal of Clinical Endocrinology and Metabolism* 83 (1998): 2773.

22. I. Zavaroni et al., "Hyperinsulinemia in a Normal Population as a Predictor of Non-Insulin-Dependent Diabetes Mellitus, Hypertension, and Coronary Heart Disease: The Barilla Factory Revisited," *Metabolism* 48, no. 8 (1999): 989–94.

23. J. P. Despres, "Hyperinsulinemia as an Independent Risk Factor for Ischemic Heart Disease," *New England Journal of Medicine* 334, no. 15 (1996): 952–57.

24. Reaven, *Syndrome X.*

25. Francois Gueyffier et al., "Antihypertensive Drugs in Very Old People: A Subgroup Meta-Analysis of Randomized Controlled Trials," *The Lancet* 353, no. 9155 (1999): 793.

26. O. Warburg, "On the Origin of Cancer Cell," *Science* 123 (1956): 309–14.

27. G. A. Santisteban et al., "Complex Versus Simple Carbohydrates and Mammary Tumors in Mice," *Biochemical Biophysics Research Community* 132, no. 3 (1985): 1174–79.

28. C. J. Moerman et al., "Dietary Sugar Intake in the Aetiology of Biliary Tract Cancer," *International Journal of Epidemiology* 22, no. 2 (1993): 207–14.

29. S. Seeley, "Diet and Breast Cancer: The Possible Connection with Sugar Consumption," *Medical Hypotheses* 11, no. 3 (1983): 319–27.

CHAPTER 4

1. Michael Mason, "Welcome Fat Back into Your Kitchen," *Health* (April 1997): 69–73.

2. Gary Evans, M.D., *Chromium Picolinate* (New York: Avery, 1996).

3. L. Hordocks, "Health Benefits of Docosahexaenoic Acid (DHA)," *Pharmaceutical Research* 40, no. 3 (1999): 211–25.

4. Johanna Budwig, M.D., *Flax Oil: As a True Aid Against Arthritis, Heart Infarction, Cancer and Other Diseases* (Canada: Apple Publishing Company, 1992).

5. Neil J. Stone, "Fish Consumption, Fish Oil, Lipids, and Coronary Heart Disease," *Circulation* 94 (1996): 2337–40.

6. D. Kromhout, E. B. Bosschieter, and C. de Lezenne Coulander, "The Inverse Relation Between Fish Consumption and 20-Year Mortality from Coronary Heart Disease," *New England Journal of Medicine* 312, no. 19 (1985): 1205–9.

7. D. S. Siscouick et al., "Dietary Intake and Cell Membrane Levels of Long-Chain n-3 Polyunsaturated Fatty Acids and the Risk of Primary Cardiac Arrest," *Journal of the American Medical Association* 274, no. 17 (1995): 1363–67.

8. J. Eritsland et al., "Effect of Dietary Supplementation with n-3 Fatty Acids on Coronary Artery Bypass Graft Patency," *American Journal of Cardiology* 77 (1996): 31–36.

9. R. L. Atkinson, "Conjugated Linoleic Acid for Altering Body Composition and Treating Obesity," in *Advances in Conjugated Linoleic Acid Research*, vol. 1 (Champaign, Ill.: AOCS Press, 1999) 348–53.

10. American Chemical Society, "CLA Could Help Control Weight, Fat, Diabetes, and Muscle Loss," American Chemical Society National Meeting News (August 20, 2000).

11. M. W. Pariza, "The Biological Activities of Conjugated Linoleic Acid," in *Advances in Conjugated Linoleic Acid Research*, vol. 1 (Champaign, Ill.: AOCS Press, 1999) 12–20.

12. Geoffrey A. Fowler, "Fighting Fat with More Fat," *U.S. News and World Report*, 4 September 2000.

13. A. E. M. Smedman and B. O. H. Vessby, "Metabolic Effect of CLA Supplementation on Human Subjects," *Clinical Nutrition Research*, Dept. of Public Health and Caring Sciences, Uppsala University.

14. M. A. Belury and J. P. Vanden Heuvel, "Modulation of Diabetes by Conjugated Linoleic Acid," in *Advances in Conjugated Linoleic Acid Research*, vol. 1 (Champaign, Ill.: AOCS Press, 1999) 404–11.

15. M. W. Pariza et al., "Conjugated Dienoic Derivatives of Linoleic Acid: Mechanism of Anticarcinogenic Effect," *Journal of Progressive Clinical Biological Research* 347 (1990): 217–21.

16. Barbara Fitch Haumann, "Conjugated Linoleic Acid Offers Research Promise," *Inform* 7, no. 2 (1996): 152, 159.

17. F. Visoli et al., "Low Density Lipoprotein Oxidation Is Inhibited in Vitro by Olive Oil Constituents," *Atherosclerosis* 117, no. 1 (1995): 25–32.

18. Scott Grundy, M.D., "Comparison of Monounsaturated Fatty Acids and Carbohydrates for Lowering Plasma Cholesterol," *The New England Journal of Medicine* 314, no. 12 (1986): 745.

19. G. E. Fraser et al., "A Possible Protective Effect of Nut Consumption on Risk of Coronary Heart Disease," *Archives of Internal Medicine* 152 (1992): 1416–24.

20. A. Wolk, Ph.D. et al., " A Prospective Study of Association of Monounsaturated Fat and Other Types of Fat with Risk of Breast Cancer," *Archives of Internal Medicine* 158 (1998): 41-45.

21. Richard A. Passwater, Ph.D., "Health Risks from Processed Foods and Trans Fats," *Whole Foods*, January 1999, 47–52.

22. Mary Enig, *Know Your Fats: The Complete Primer for Understanding the Nutrition of Fats, Oils, and Cholesterol* (Silver Springs, Md.: Bethesda Press, 2000), 85

CHAPTER 7

1. U.S. Senate Doc. 264, 1936.
2. Paul Bergner, *The Healing Power of Minerals* (Rocklin, Calif.: Prima Publishing, 1997), 59–61.
3. M. Seelig, "Magnesium Requirements in Human Nutrition," *Journal of Medical Society* 79, no. 11 (1982): 849–50.
4. J. S. Parker et al., "Selenium Supplementation and Cancer Rates," *Journal of the American Medical Association* 277, no. 11 (1997): 880–81.
5. G. N. Schrauzer et al., "Soil Levels of Selenium and Related Cancer Incidence," *Bioinorganic Chemistry* 7 (1977): 23.
6. M. A. Beck, "Selenium and Host Defense Towards Viruses," *Proceedings of the Nutrition Society* 58, no. 3 (1999): 707–11.
7. W. J. Walsh, "Treatment of Mental Illness and Behavior Disorders," *Health Research Institute Newsletter,* 17 November 1997.
8. F. J. Antonawich, S. M. Fiore, and J. N. Davis, "The Effects of a Lipoic Acid/Palladium Complex on Hippocampal Progenitor Cells," *Society for Neuroscience Abstract* 857-10, no. 24 (1998): 2161.

CHAPTER 8

1. Peter J. D'Adamo, M.D., *Eat Right for Your Type* (New York: Putnam, 1996).

CHAPTER 9

1. Marian Burros, "Losing Count of Calories as Plates Fill Up," *New York Times,* 2 April 1997.

RESOURCES

PRODUCTS

As a convenience for my readers and clients, Uni Key Health Systems has been the main distributor of my products, books, and services over the years. Uni Key carries several of the formulas I recommend, including the copper-free Female Multiple, iron-free Male Multiple, Weight-Loss Formula, L-carnitine, Co-Q10, Super Max EPA, GLA, Super GI Cleanse, and Evening Primrose. Be sure to call for a catalog of all the latest products. You may also order all of my books through Uni Key.

Uni Key Health Systems
P.O. Box 7168
Bozeman, MT 59771
1-800-888-4353
www.unikeyhealth.com

BOOKS

Books by Ann Louise Gittleman

Before the Change (HarperSanFrancisco, ISBN 0-06-2515367-3)
The first complete do-it-yourself program for managing perimenopause
—the period of about ten years leading up to menopause—with
proven techniques for understanding and controlling its symptoms
without powerful drugs or hormone treatments.

Beyond Pritikin (Bantam Books, ISBN 0-553-57400-0)
This book tells you everything you always wanted to know (but were
afraid to ask) about curbing those crazy carbohydrates, fats, cholesterol, triglycerides, and fat-burning nutrients. A total nutrition program for weight loss, longevity, and good health.

Eat Fat, Lose Weight (Keats Publishing, ISBN 0-87983-966-X)
Fat is your best friend when it comes to weight loss. This book talks
about the right fats from the omega 3, 6, and 9 families contained in
such foods as flaxseed, nuts, seeds, evening primrose oil, avocadoes,
and olive oil and how they are fundamental to our health and vitality.

Eat Fat, Lose Weight Cookbook (Keats Publishing, ISBN 0-658-01220-7)
Say farewell to the cuisine of deprivation and introduce a whole new
cuisine of celebration. You'll develop a brand-new attitude toward
eating, one that focuses on the amazing omega fats—fats that not
only brim with flavor, but also are bursting with health benefits.

The Living Beauty Detox Program (HarperSanFrancisco,
ISBN 0-06251-628-0)
The right nutrition, internal cleansing, and hormonal harmony are
the pathways to attaining natural beauty and vitality. This book
presents detailed beauty tips for different life stages, strategies for
detoxifying your emotions, and chemicals to avoid in cosmetics and
household products.

How to Stay Young and Healthy in a Toxic World (Keats Publishing, ISBN 0-87983-907-4)

This book explores the four greatest hidden threats to health: sugar, parasites, heavy metals, and radiation. Learn how to avoid the toxic invaders from your life and find out the natural and even surprising solutions for the toxins that surround us in food, water, and our homes and workplaces.

Get the Salt Out (Crown, ISBN 0-517-88654-57)

This is *the* essential book for those who need to reduce salt intake due to hypertension and risk of stroke! *Get the Salt Out* provides the tips, menu plans, and recipes to help you enjoy real foods again and create meals that both your taste buds and your body can truly savor.

Get the Sugar Out (Crown, ISBN 0-517-88653-7)

Sugar has been connected with no less than sixty ailments, including weight gain, cardiovascular disease, cancer, adult-onset diabetes, and impaired immunity. Fortunately, this book makes it easy to get the sugar out with indispensable tips and fifty delicious recipes. My low-sugar plan is easy to incorporate into your diet, yet filled with flavor and variety.

Guess What Came to Dinner? (Avery, ISBN 1-58333-096-8)

A newly revised and updated edition of an authoritative book on parasitic infections—their detection, treatment, and cure. This book offers practical advice to parasite-proof your food and water and explains breakthrough methods of detection, antiparasitic treatments, and herbal cures.

Overcoming Parasites: What You Need to Know (Avery, ISBN 0-89529-983-6)

How to parasite-proof your diet and your lifestyle. In easy-to-understand language, this book clearly explains what parasites are, why they are harmful, and how they are spread. It also provides information on diagnosing, treating, and, most importantly, preventing parasites.

Super Nutrition for Men (Avery, ISBN 0-89529-954-2)
Authoritative guide full of practical advice to help men reduce their risk of succumbing to such common male ailments as heart disease, cancer, hypertension, and stroke. Ladies, this book is *not* just for guys.

Super Nutrition for Menopause (Avery, ISBN 0-89529-877-5)
Learn how nutritional deficiencies can throw off the body's natural mineral balance and aggravate menopausal symptoms, and how a proper diet and vitamin regimen along with the right amount of exercise can ease the discomforts of menopause.

Super Nutrition for Women (Bantam Books, ISBN 0-553-35328-4)
The perfect book for women in their twenties and thirties who want to learn how to lose weight, combat PMS and yeast infections, and strengthen their immune systems. Learn how to reprogram your harmful eating habits to reenergize and recharge your body.

Why Am I Always So Tired? (HarperSanFrancisco, ISBN 0-06251-569-1)
A revitalizing guide that provides solid answers to the question "Why am I always so tired?" This book shows how simple dietary changes can dramatically improve the way you feel and discusses the overlooked connection between exhaustion and a copper/zinc imbalance in our bodies.

Your Body Knows Best (Pocket Books, ISBN 0-671-87591-4)
Here is an approach that meets your body's special needs right now. Your customized diet is determined by your ancestry and genetic heritage, blood type, and metabolism. This is a revolutionary eating plan that helps you achieve your optimal weight and energy level for life.

ADDITIONAL HELP ON THE WEB

www.annlouise.com. If you would like to see what I am up to, catch up with my schedule, book me for a lecture, make an appointment for a consultation, or join my mailing list, please visit my Web site.

www.fatsforhealth.com. This is a comprehensive online guide for essential fatty acid information and news. You can get up-to-date data, articles, and news about EFAs in health, nutrition, beauty, disease treatment, and even pet care. This Web site tells you everything and more than you wanted to know about healthy fats.

www.zonebalance.com. At this site you can order online the Zone Balance software, mentioned in Chapter 10, to help keep your meals and snacks within the right parameters. The software is easy to use and based on the 100-calorie food block concept, originated by Barry Sears, and currently used by many others. The Web site also offers links to other 40/30/30-related information.

www.drsears.com. The best Zone Web site out there by far. Dr. Barry Sears provides lifestyle and update news tips on the Zone as well as information on preparing Zone-certified meals, research, resources, and recipes. A Zone cruise, anyone?

PARTNERS FOR WOMEN'S HEALTH

Dedicating my career to women's health has been tremendously rewarding. But I wanted to help women even more, so I began searching for a venue to accomplish that deep-seated desire. I knew that if women partnered together, we could promote the health of women to even higher levels. That belief prompted me to create a nonprofit organization called Key to Health.

The Key to Health Foundation is committed to bettering women's health by creating a platform that will empower them at every transition of their lives, setting a nutritional revolution in motion that will reach out to future generations as well. To achieve this goal, Key to Health partners with other organizations that parallel its mission, principles, and holistic philosophy. It is through these combined, dedicated efforts that Key to Health plans to one day fund research studies for breakthrough natural remedies, responding to twenty-first-century health challenges. Eventually the keys to healing, longevity, and well-being will be readily available to women of every age.

If you would like to learn more about Key to Health or how you can become a partner in my quest to promote women's health, please write to me for an introductory packet:

Key to Health Foundation
P.O. Box 882
Bozeman, MT 59771

ABOUT THE AUTHOR

ANN LOUISE GITTLEMAN, N.D., M.S., C.N.S., IS ONE OF THE most respected and dynamic nutritionists in America today, continually breaking new ground in both traditional and holistic health. After graduating with a bachelor of arts degree from Connecticut College, Ann Louise attained a master's degree in nutrition education from Columbia University. She later went on to attain a doctor of naturopathy degree. In 1993, Ann Louise became a certified nutrition specialist through the American College of Nutrition.

Hailed as the "first lady of nutrition" and respected as one of the most knowledgeable nutritionists in America, Ann Louise travels internationally as a speaker and consultant. She also regularly contributes to national radio, television, magazines, and newspapers. Her articles, insights, and books have enlightened the public on a variety of health-related topics. Countless major magazines and newspapers, including *Publisher's Weekly, Newsweek, Harper's Bazaar, Family Circle, New Woman, McCall's, Fitness, Black Elegance, Good*

Housekeeping, Self, Women's World, First for Women, Parade Magazine, the *New York Times,* and the *Los Angeles Times,* have quoted Ann Louise or featured her work. She has also appeared on ABC's *Good Morning America,* MSNBC's *Home Page, Fox News Live,* and the popular *Ainsley Harriott Show.*

Ann Louise is the prolific, bestselling author of nearly twenty books, including *Beyond Pritikin; Super Nutrition for Women; Super Nutrition for Menopause; Eat Fat, Lose Weight;* and the *Eat Fat, Lose Weight Cookbook.* Her latest book, *The Fat Flush Plan,* will be out in 2002.

INDEX

adult-onset diabetes. *See* type 2
    diabetes
advanced glycosylation end prod-
    ucts (AGEs), 17, 18
aging, and excess blood sugar,
    17–18
alpha-linoleic acid (ALA), xiv
Alzheimer's disease, 30
American Heart Association, 28
American Journal of Cardiology, 30
amino acids, 42
ancestry, 59–60
Archives of Internal Medicine, 34
athletes, and diet, xi, 3
Atkins, Robert, 18
Atkinson, Richard, 32
attention deficit hyperactivity
    disorder (ADHD), xiv, 30

Belury, Martha, 33
Beyond Pritikin, ix, xiii
blood sugar levels, xiii, 14–15.

See also glucose; sugar
and aging, 17–18
and dietary fat, 2
and high-carbohydrate diets,
    xiii, 2
and insulin, 14
low, 18
stabilizing, 2, 3, 31, 41
blood type, 63–65
Borg scale, xi
boron, 57
Brand-Miller, Jennie, 12
Budwig, Johanna, 30
Burros, Marian, 69

calcium, 52
cancer, xv, 24–25, 33, 34
Candida albicans, xv
carbohydrate loading, 3
carbohydrates, 2, 9–25. *See also*
    high-carbohydrate diet
complex, x, 10

139